# Bridging Science and Practical Appliance in Resistance Training

*Edited by Daniel A. Marinho, Pedro Forte, Maria Cirilo-Sousa and Henrique P. Neiva*

Published in London, United Kingdom

Bridging Science and Practical Appliance in Resistance Training
http://dx.doi.org/10.5772/intechopen.104335
Edited by Daniel A. Marinho, Pedro Forte, Maria Cirilo-Sousa and Henrique P. Neiva

Contributors
Mijin Kim, Azzam Alarab, Nadeen Taqatqa, Abrão José Melhem Junior, David Livingstone Alves Figueiredo, Miguel Morita Fernandes-Silva, Endang Ernandini, William Giovanni Mulyanaga, Alison Morag Murray, Kristy Howells, Pamela Murray, Aly Matejka, Francisco Saavedra



First published in London, United Kingdom, 2023 by IntechOpen
IntechOpen is the global imprint of INTECHOPEN LIMITED, registered in England and Wales, registration number: 11086078, 5 Princes Gate Court, London, SW7 2QJ, United Kingdom

British Library Cataloguing-in-Publication Data
A catalogue record for this book is available from the British Library

Additional hard and PDF copies can be obtained from orders@intechopen.com

Bridging Science and Practical Appliance in Resistance Training
Edited by Daniel A. Marinho, Pedro Forte, Maria Cirilo-Sousa and Henrique P. Neiva
p. cm.
Print ISBN 978-1-83768-550-9
Online ISBN 978-1-83768-551-6
eBook (PDF) ISBN 978-1-83768-552-3

# Meet the editors

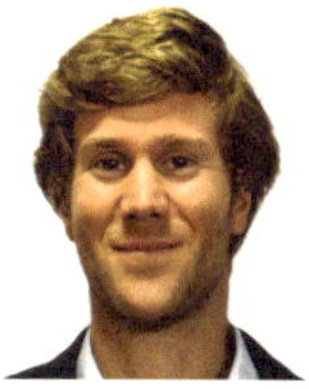

Daniel Almeida Marinho has been an associate professor at the University of Beira Interior (UBI), Portugal since 2008 and the director of the Ph.D. sports sciences course since 2013. He obtained a degree in Sport and Physical Education at the University of Porto in 2004, a Ph.D. in Sport Sciences at the University of Trás-os-Montes e Alto Douro (UTAD) in 2009, and a habilitation in Sport Sciences at UBI in 2013. He has supervised twenty graduate theses, twenty MD theses, and ten PhD theses. He has published more than 150 academic titles, including ten books and book chapters, 60 articles in SCI journals, 70 articles in peer-reviewed indexed international journals, and 10 articles in peer-reviewed indexed national journals. He has participated in the organisation of fifteen national and international scientific meetings and has been a member of several Ph.D. and MD juries. Since 2013, he has been working with the Portuguese Swimming Federation, where he is responsible for coaching courses and coordinates the Evaluation and Control Training Centre.

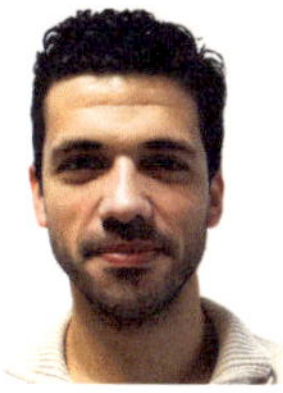

Pedro Miguel Gomes Forte obtained a degree in Sports in 2012 and a master's degree in Exercise and Health in 2014, both from the Polytechnic Institute of Bragança, Portugal. He completed his Ph.D. in Sports Sciences at the University of Beira Interior (UBI), Portugal, in 2018. He is a coordinator professor at the Instituto Superior de Ciências Educativas do Douro, Portugal, and a guest professor at the Polytechnic Institute of Bragança. He is also a basketball and football coach. The focus of his sports science research is biomechanics, particularly prevalence, posture, youth, asymmetries, risk factors, football, training, analysis, performance, computational fluid dynamics, aerodynamics, drag, hydrodynamics, and kinematics.

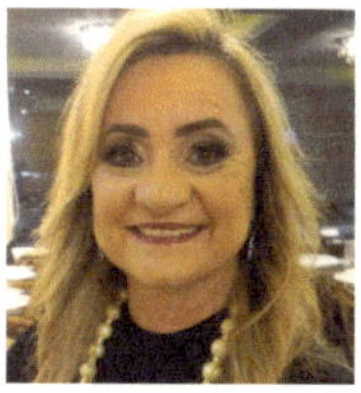

Maria S. Cirilo-Sousa is an assistant professor (Ph.D.) in the Department of Physical Education – Associate Graduate Program in Physical Education at the Federal University of Paraíba. Her research interests involve the resistance exercise with blood flow restriction with different objectives in different populations.

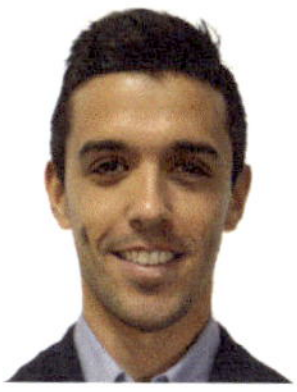

Henrique Neiva obtained his Ph.D. in Sport Sciences at the University of Beira Interior (UBI), Portugal, in 2015, supported by a grant from the Science and Technology Foundation. He has more than fifty scientific publications to his credit and has published several peer-reviewed papers in high-ranked journals. A former international swimmer and Level 3 coach, Dr. Neiva's original academic interest was in training and competition, specifically swimming. His interest in exercise and health, and specifically in technological development, has emerged in the last two years due to his recent post-doctoral research with the NanoSTIMA project at the University of Trás-os-Montes and Alto Douro, Research Centre for Sports Sciences, Health Sciences and Human Development (UTAD/CIDESD). He has been a member of the CIDESD since 2015.

# Contents

# Preface

This book is a comprehensive guide for athletes, trainers, and enthusiasts alike, delving into the intricate science behind resistance training and its profound impact on athletic development. As the pursuit of excellence in sports continues to evolve, the significance of resistance training has grown exponentially. It is no longer viewed as a mere ancillary component but rather as a foundational pillar in achieving peak performance. This book seeks to unravel the mysteries surrounding resistance training, providing a comprehensive understanding of its physiological, biomechanical, and psychological intricacies.

This book highlights the role of resistance exercise in injury prevention and rehabilitation, showcasing the profound impact it can have on musculoskeletal health and overall well-being. We examine the interplay between strength training and various sports, uncovering sport-specific training protocols tailored to individual needs. As such, the book presents a wide range of themes and it is organized into three sections: "Children", "Medicine", and "Ageing".

The first section includes two chapters. Chapter 1, "A Study on the Relationship between Health and Physical Fitness and School Life of Children", investigates how the health and physical fitness of children impact their school life. It explores the connection between overall well-being and academic performance, social interactions, and behavior. The findings could inform educational policies and promote the integration of health and fitness programs in schools. Chapter 2, "Accessible Resistance Movement Experiences for Elementary Students and Educators" highlights the importance of resistance movement in sedentary students and educators and recommends programs for active living time in school.

The second section includes three chapters. Chapter 3, "Resistance Training is Medicine: Stay Active and Reap the Reward Live in your Life!", analyzes the benefits of resistance training during the life cycle and how it promotes better quality of life. Chapter 4, "Resistance Exercises for Musculoskeletal Disorders", examines the relationship between strength levels and resistance exercises for different musculoskeletal problems, with a focus on functional fitness. The chapter alsofocuses on resistance exercises as a therapeutic approach for musculoskeletal disorders. It discusses the benefits of resistance training in improving strength, flexibility, and function. The chapter also explores various resistance exercise techniques and their applications in managing and rehabilitating musculoskeletal conditions. Finally, Chapter 5, "Guidelines for Prenatal and Postpartum Resistance Training" highlights the importance of resistance training during pregnancy and after birth. It highlights the training's benefits and discusses how women can benefit from it in terms of quality of life and well-being.

The third section includes two chapters. Chapter 6, "Strength Training, Quality of Life, and Health in Elderly" and Chapter 7, "Functional Capacity in Advanced Older

Adults" examine the functional capacity of older adults. They delve into the physical and cognitive changes that occur with aging and their impact on daily functioning. The chapters explore strategies and interventions aimed at maintaining or improving functional abilities in this population, enhancing their overall quality of life.

While rooted in science, this book also recognizes the artistry and passion that define the world of sports and exercise. It celebrates the dedication, discipline, and perseverance required to excel in athletic pursuits. Through captivating case studies, anecdotes, and firsthand accounts, we witness the transformative power of resistance training, not only in physical performance but also in fostering mental resilience and determination.

**Daniel A. Marinho**
Associate Professor,
Department of Sports Sciences,
University of Beira Interior,
Covilhã, Portugal

**Pedro Forte**
Coordinator Professor,
Department of Sports,
Higher Institute of Educational Sciences of the Douro,
Penafiel, Portugal

**Henrique P. Neiva**
Department of Sports Sciences,
University of Beira Interior,
Covilhã, Portugal

**Maria Cirilo-Sousa**
Physical Education/LABOCINE,
Federal University of Paraíba,
João Pessoa, Brazil

Section 1

# Children

Chapter 1

# A Study on the Relationship between Health and Physical Fitness and School Life of Children

*Mijin Kim*


## Abstract

In this study, in order to clarify the relationship between health and physical strength, athletic capability, school life, and lifestyles, we collated the results of physical fitness tests with questionnaire surveys of 102 elementary school fifth-grade males and females. In the school life aspect, children who scored high on the physical fitness test, like Physical Education, enjoy learning, play well with friends while in the lifestyle aspect, they clean up their surroundings and rooms, study even without being told and there is a tendency for them to make their own plan. In addition, it was confirmed that children with high physical fitness test scores were in good condition, such as being healthy every day and hardly getting sick. On the other hand, in relation to the physical fitness test scores and the body shape by BMI, there were many high scorers among the children whose body figure was standard. These results suggest that physical fitness and athletic capability are related to children's school life and health, and that high physical fitness has a positive impact on children's school life and health.


**Keywords:** physique, physical fitness, school life, health, elementary school student

## 1. Introduction

Physical strength is the source of human activity and an important element of "the power to live" such as abundant humanity, the ability to learn by oneself and the ability to think for themselves [1, 2].

In recent years, changes in the social environment and lifestyle have led to great changes in the environment surrounding children. There is a decrease in walking opportunities for children due to the development of transportation, the neglect of adults to disregard children's play and sports, a decrease in helping children's housework, and the development of information equipment, etc.

As a result, children's human relationships become weak, and there are fewer opportunities to have more friends and to move their bodies [1, 2].

Along with this, the current physical strength of children around 1985, has been declining over the long term in all ages, such as their running power, throwing power and gripping power, etc. [3].

Also, recently, the bipolarization of physical strength between children who are actively engaged in exercise and sports and those who lack exercise has been pointed out [4]. Children's lack of exercise is not just a decline in physical strength, but also has an adverse effect on the improvement of mental and physical health [5].

In a questionnaire survey on children's experience activities conducted by the Ministry of Education, Culture, Sports, Science, and Technology in 1998, a total of 33% of elementary school second graders answered that they "often" or "sometimes" feel tired on a daily basis and it is reported that it reaches 60% in the second grade of junior high school [6].

Also, there are quite a few children who have stress in their school life resulting in disturbed lifestyles such as spending a considerable amount of time studying at school, studying at cram school or at home, having insufficient sleeping time, being unable to sleep at night, being easy to get tired, having no desire for breakfast, wanting to speak out loud somehow and being frustrated with nothing.

Furthermore, disruption of children's lifestyles can have a negative impact on reduced energy and motivation and a lack of concentration [7]. It may be said that the lack of exercise in children greatly affects the development of their strength and growth.

Therefore, it is thought to be extremely important to examine athletic ability and physical strength which is the basis for living.

Up to now, many research endeavors have been conducted from various angles to solve this problem, and various improvement measures have been tried on how children's physical fitness and exercise capacity are related to school life and lifestyle and it is deemed necessary to conduct further verification.

Therefore, the purpose of this study is to examine in detail the physical strength and athletic capability of elementary school students such as running ability, jumping ability, throwing ability and endurance and to clarify the relationship between health and physical strength, athletic capability, school life and lifestyle.

## 2. Method

### 2.1 Participants

A self-administered questionnaire survey was conducted for fifth graders of a public elementary school in Tokyo. There were 47 boys and 55 females for a total of 102 respondents.

### 2.2 Investigation contents

#### *2.2.1 Fitness test*

The physical fitness tests conducted at the school were: muscle strength: grip strength, muscle endurance: upper body, flexibility: sit and reach, agility: repeated sideways jump, whole body endurance: 20 m shuttle run, speed, running ability: 50 m run, muscle power, jumping ability: standing long jump, skill, and muscle power and throwing power: softball throwing. The results were recorded on a 10-point scale according to the score table for each item set by the Sports Bureau of the Ministry of Education, Culture, Sports, Science, and Technology (MEXT). In addition, the total result was calculated by adding the scores of each item. Based on the comprehensive evaluation criteria table of the new physical fitness test, comprehensive evaluation was obtained in five stages from A to E. A and B were set to "high," C was set to "standard," while D and E were set to "low."

#### *2.2.2 Figure*

At the school, the BMI was calculated from the height and weight of body measurements. Based on that, we used Kato's [8] age-specific BMI percentile curves up to 18 years old by classifying obesity, standard, and lean body types. The body type is determined by setting the 10 to 90 percentile value of each age in the BMI percentile curve as "standard" (15.0 to 18.5). In addition, "lean" is defined as less than this range, and "obesity" is defined as exceeding this range.

#### *2.2.3 Analysis method*

The physical fitness test and body type and each question item were examined by gender. Furthermore, we examined the relationship between physical strength tests and school life and health; and between physical strength tests and body types.

All analyzes were performed with SPSS19.0 for Windows, with a significance level of 5%. The $\chi 2$ test was used to test the ratio bias, and the unmatched t-test was used to test the difference between the average values of BMI and physical strength test results.

## 3. Result

### 3.1 Gender differences in physical characteristics and physical strength/athletic capability test results

In terms of physical characteristics, the sitting height was $75.6 \pm 3.6$ for boys and $77.3 \pm 3.7$ for girls, with girls significantly higher than boys ($p < 0.05$) (**Table 1**). In the physical strength test, for softball throwing: the score was $21.72 \pm 6.97$ m for boys and $11.87 \pm 3.32$ m for girls ($p < 0.001$). In repeated sideways jumps, the score was $36.36 \pm 7.05$ for boys and $33.51 \pm 33.51$ for girls ($p < 0.05$). In the 20 m shuttle run, the boys had $43.60 \pm 20.84$ times while the girls were $30.98 \pm 12.77$ times ($p < 0.001$).

On the other hand, in the sit and reach test the score was $31.00 \pm 7.94$ cm for boys and $38.00 \pm 8.73$ cm for girls, with girls showing significantly higher results compared to boys ($p < 0.000$). The overall fitness test score was slightly higher for girls than for boys, but there was no significant difference. In addition, boys have low scores and little higher standard scores, while girls had slightly higher scores.

### 3.2 Gender differences in physical fitness and athletic capability test evaluation

The percentage of "high" scores for both boys and girls exceeded 50%, but the percentage of girls was slightly higher than that of boys. However, the percentage of "low" scores was slightly higher for boys than for girls, but no significant difference was observed (**Table 2**).

| | Boys (11) | | | | | Girls (11) | | | | | 95% confidence interval for difference | | |
|---|---|---|---|---|---|---|---|---|---|---|---|---|---|
| | n | m | sd | Minimum value | Maximum value | n | m | sd | Minimum value | Maximum value | Minimum limit | Maximum value | Significance |
| Physical characteristic | | | | | | | | | | | | | |
| Height (cm) | 47 | 139.8 | 6.9 | 122.5 | 153.3 | 55 | 142.2 | 6.5 | 124.8 | 154.7 | −4.956 | 0.319 | 0.526 |
| Weight (kg) | 47 | 35.5 | 9.3 | 21.3 | 72.0 | 55 | 34.4 | 6.0 | 22.6 | 50.2 | −2.049 | 4.252 | 0.026* |
| Sit height (cm) | 47 | 75.6 | 3.6 | 65.3 | 83.2 | 55 | 77.3 | 3.7 | 68.0 | 84.3 | −3.192 | −0.298 | 0.989 |
| BMI (kg/m$^2$) | 47 | 18.0 | 3.5 | 14.2 | 32.6 | 55 | 16.9 | 2.0 | 13.5 | 22.0 | −0.042 | 2.131 | 0.007** |
| Physical strength test | | | | | | | | | | | | | |
| Grip strength (kg) | 47 | 17.7 | 3.3 | 10 | 27 | 55 | 18.0 | 4.0 | 8 | 27 | −1.792 | 1.153 | 0.062 |
| Upper body development (times) | 47 | 20.3 | 4.1 | 11 | 28 | 55 | 19.9 | 3.4 | 10 | 27 | −1.107 | 1.836 | 0.226 |
| Sit and reach (cm) | 47 | 31.0 | 7.9 | 5 | 43 | 55 | 38.0 | 8.7 | 18 | 57 | −10.301 | −3.699 | 0.541 |
| Repeated horizontal jump (points) | 47 | 36.4 | 7.1 | 18 | 48 | 55 | 33.5 | 5.9 | 15 | 43 | 0.312 | 5.393 | 0.150 |
| 20 m shuttle run (times) | 47 | 43.6 | 20.8 | 5 | 91 | 54 | 31.0 | 12.8 | 12 | 75 | 5.638 | 19.591 | 0.001*** |
| 50 m race (seconds) | 47 | 9.7 | 2.3 | 8.1 | 20.1 | 54 | 9.4 | 0.8 | 7.9 | 12 | −0.467 | 0.927 | 0.035* |
| Standing long jump (cm) | 47 | 147.4 | 20.9 | 89 | 187 | 55 | 145.8 | 18.6 | 100 | 185 | −6.144 | 9.383 | 0.657 |
| Throw a ball (m) | 47 | 21.7 | 7.0 | 11 | 38 | 55 | 11.9 | 3.3 | 6 | 23 | 7.632 | 12.069 | 0.001*** |
| Physical strength general score | 47 | 57.6 | 9.4 | 37 | 76 | 55 | 59.7 | 8.6 | 41 | 83 | −5.655 | 1.440 | 0.595 |

*BMI: Body Mass Index.*
*: $p < .05$. **: $p < .01$. ***: $p < .001$.

**Table 1.**
*Gender differences in physical characteristics and physical fitness test results.*

| | | Boys | Girls | Total | Significance |
|---|---|---|---|---|---|
| Comprehensive evaluation of physical fitness | low | 9 (19.1) | 7 (12.7) | 16 (15.7) | 0.523 |
| | standard | 13 (27.7) | 13 (23.6) | 26 (25.5) | |
| | high | 25 (53.2) | 35 (63.6) | 60 (58.8) | |
| | Total | 47 (100.0) | 55 (100.0) | 102 (100.0) | |

*N (%).*

**Table 2.**
*Gender differences in physical fitness test evaluation.*

### 3.3 Gender differences in school life aspect, lifestyle aspect, health aspect, degree of obesity, and sleep time

At school, many children answered that they were having fun. In particular, a high percentage of male respondents answered the items "I like physical education classes" and "play well with friends when playing" compared to girls. Compared with boys, girls responded more frequently to items such as "school is fun", "study is fun", and "has good friends" (**Table 3**). In terms of lifestyle habits, boys and girls accounted for more than 70% of the children who answered "yes" in the "staying at home alone" item. For most items, more children answered "No" than "Yes".

In the items "I have decided what I want to be in the future" and "I have something I want to do when I grow up" ($p < 0.01$), the percentage of "Yes" for girls was higher than that for boys.

| | | Boys | Girls | Total | Significance |
|---|---|---|---|---|---|
| School life | Is school fun? | | | | |
| | Yes, it's fun. | 33 (70.2) | 41 (74.5) | 74 (72.5) | 0.423 |
| | No, it is not. | 6 (12.8) | 3 (5.5) | 9 (8.8) | |
| | Neither | 8 (17.0) | 11 (20.0) | 19 (18.6) | |
| | Total | 47 (100.0) | 55 (100.0) | 102 (100.0) | |
| | Is studying at school fun? | | | | |
| | Yes, it is. | 28 (59.6) | 43 (78.2) | 71 (69.6) | 0.080 |
| | No, I do not. | 8 (17.0) | 3 (5.5) | 11 (10.8) | |
| | Neither | 11 (23.4) | 9 (16.4) | 20 (19.6) | |
| | Total | 47 (100.0) | 55 (100.0) | 102 (100.0) | |
| | Do you like school physical education? | | | | |
| | Yes, I do. | 42 (89.4) | 45 (81.8) | 87 (85.3) | 0.430 |
| | No, I do not. | 1 (2.1) | 4 (7.3) | 5 (4.9) | |
| | Neither | 4 (8.5) | 6 (10.9) | 10 (9.8) | |
| | Total | 47 (100.0) | 55 (100.0) | 102 (100.0) | |

| | | Boys | Girls | Total | Significance |
|---|---|---|---|---|---|
| | Do you have close friends? | | | | |
| | Yes, I do. | 46 (97.9) | 54 (98.2) | 100 (98.0) | 0.911 |
| | No, I do not. | 1 (2.1) | 1 (1.8) | 2 (2.0) | |
| | Total | 47 (100.0) | 55100.0 | 102 (100.0) | |
| | Do you often play with friends during the playing time at school? | | | | |
| | Yes, I do. | 39 (83.0) | 42 (76.4) | 81 (79.4) | 0.669 |
| | Sometimes | 7 (14.9) | 12 (21.8) | 19 (18.6) | |
| | No, I do not. | 1 (2.1) | 1 (1.8) | 2 (2.0) | |
| | Total | 47 (100.0) | 55 (100.0) | 102 (100.0) | |
| Lifestyle aspects | I get up alone in the morning. | 22 (46.8) | 27 (49.1) | 49 (48.0) | 0.818 |
| | I stay at home alone. | 33 (70.2) | 38 (69.1) | 71 (69.6) | 0.902 |
| | I clean up my surroundings and my room. | 20 (42.6) | 27 (49.1) | 47 (46.1) | 0.509 |
| | I stop playing when the set time comes even during the play. | 23 (48.9) | 27 (49.1) | 50 (49.0) | 0.988 |
| | I decide what TV programs I want but do not watch constantly. | 14 (29.8) | 18 (32.7) | 32 (31.4) | 0.750 |
| | I make plans and study even if not told. | 15 (31.9) | 22 (40.0) | 37 (36.3) | 0.397 |
| | I decide what I want to be in the future | 21 (44.7) | 33 (60.0) | 54 (52.9) | 0.122 |
| | There are things I want to try when I grow up. | 19 (40.4) | 37 (67.3) | 56 (54.9) | 0.007** |
| Health | I feel heavy and maybe tired | | | | |
| | Often | 4 (10.5) | 4 (9.1) | 8 (9.8) | 0.514 |
| | Sometimes | 22 (57.9) | 19 (43.2) | 41 (50.0) | |
| | Not much | 9 (23.7) | 15 (34.1) | 24 (29.3) | |
| | Not at all | 3 (7.9) | 6 (13.6) | 9 (11.0) | |
| | Total | 38 (100.0) | 44 (100.0) | 82 (100.0) | |
| | I spend time well every day. | | | | |
| | Very well | 17 (44.7) | 24 (54.5) | 41 (50.0) | 0.247 |
| | Healthy | 19 (50.0) | 20 (45.5) | 39 (47.6) | |
| | Not fine at all | 2 (5.3) | 0 0 | 2 (2.4) | |
| | Total | 38 (100.0) | 44 (100.0) | 82 (100.0) | |
| | There's a time that I feel sick | | | | |
| | Often | 2 (5.4) | 1 (2.3) | 3 (3.7) | 0.660 |
| | Sometimes | 15 (40.5) | 21 (47.7) | 36 (44.4) | |
| | Almost never | 20 (54.1) | 22 (50.0) | 42 (51.9) | |
| | Total | 37 (100.0) | 44 (100.0) | 81 (100.0) | |

| | | Boys | Girls | Total | Significance |
|---|---|---|---|---|---|
| Degree of obesity | Slender | 5 (10.6) | 9 (16.4) | 14 (13.7) | 0.434 |
| | Standard | 29 (61.7) | 36 (65.5) | 65 (63.7) | |
| | Obese | 13 (27.7) | 10 (18.2) | 23 (22.5) | |
| | Total | 47 (100.0) | 55 (100.0) | 102 (100.0) | |
| Sleep time | Sleep time on weekdays | | | | |
| | More than 6 hours but less than 7 hours | 5 (13.2) | 2 (4.5) | 7 (8.5) | 0.340 |
| | More than 7 hours but less than 8 hours | 10 (26.3) | 15 (34.1) | 25 (30.5) | |
| | More than 8 hours but less than 9 hours | 13 (34.2) | 19 (43.2) | 32 (39.0) | |
| | More than 9 hours but less than 10 hours | 10 (26.3) | 7 (15.9) | 17 (20.7) | |
| | More than 10 hours | 0 0 | 1 (2.3) | 1 (1.2) | |
| | Total | 38 (100.0) | 44 (100.0) | 82 (100.0) | |
| | Sleep time on holidays | | | | |
| | More than 6 hours but less than 7 hours | 2 (5.4) | 2 (4.8) | 4 (5.1) | 0.080 |
| | More than 7 hours but less than 8 hours | 3 (8.1) | 7 (16.7) | 10 (12.7) | |
| | More than 8 hours but less than 9 hours | 21 (56.8) | 11 (26.2) | 32 (40.5) | |
| | More than 9 hours but less than 10 hours | 6 (16.2) | 14 (33.3) | 20 (25.3) | |
| | More than 10 hours | 5 (13.5) | 8 (19.0) | 13 (16.5) | |
| | Total | 37 (100.0) | 42 (100.0) | 79 (100.0) | |

**Table 3.**
*Gender differences in school life aspect, lifestyle aspect, health aspect, degree of obesity, and sleep time.*

In terms of health, most of the boys and girls were "very well" and "healthy" in the item "I spend time well every day". On the other hand, there were about 50% of children were feeling heavy or tired and sometimes get sick.

In terms of obesity, the percentage of leanness was slightly higher for girls than for boys, and the percentage of obesity was 27.7% for boys and 18.2% for girls, which was higher for boys. In the sleeping hours on weekdays, both boys and girls had a high rate of 8 hours to less than 9 hours. On holidays, boys had the highest rate of 8 hours to less than 9 hours, and girls had a slightly higher rate of 9 hours to less than 10 hours.

### 3.4 Relationship between physical strength and athletic capability test evaluation and school life

Many children with high physical strength and athletic capability test evaluations answered that they enjoyed studying ($p < 0.05$), liked physical education at school (p

| | Low | Standard | High | Total | Significance |
|---|---|---|---|---|---|
| Is school fun? | | | | | |
| Yes, it is. | 9 (56.3) | 17 (65.4) | 48 (80.0) | 74 (72.5) | 0.071 |
| No, it is not. | 4 (25.0) | 3 (11.5) | 2 (3.3) | 9 (8.8) | |
| Neither | 3 (18.8) | 6 (23.1) | 10 (16.7) | 19 (18.6) | |
| Total | 16 (100.0) | 26 (100.0) | 60 (100.0) | 102 (100.0) | |
| Is studying at school fun? | | | | | |
| Yes, it is. | 7 (43.8) | 17 (65.4) | 47 (78.3) | 71 (69.6) | 0.042* |
| No, it is not. | 3 (18.8) | 5 (19.2) | 3 (5.0) | 11 (10.8) | |
| Neither | 6 (37.5) | 4 (15.4) | 10 (16.7) | 20 (19.6) | |
| Total | 16 (100.0) | 26 (100.0) | 60 (100.0) | 102 (100.0) | |
| Do you often play with friends well during the playing time at school? | | | | | |
| Yes, I do. | 8 (50.0) | 20 (76.9) | 53 (88.3) | 81 (79.4) | 0.001*** |
| Sometimes | 6 (37.5) | 6 (23.1) | 7 (11.7) | 19 (18.6) | |
| No, I do not. | 2 (12.5) | 0 0 | 0 0 | 2 (2.0) | |
| Total | 16100.0 | 26 (100.0) | 60 (100.0) | 102 (100.0) | |
| Do you like physical education of the school? | | | | | |
| Yes, I do. | 10 (62.5) | 20 (76.9) | 57 (95.0) | 87 (85.3) | 0.003** |
| No, I do not. | 3 (18.8) | 1 (3.8) | 1 (1.7) | 5 (4.9) | |
| Neither | 3 (18.8) | 5 (19.2) | 2 (3.3) | 10 (9.8) | |
| Total | 16 (100.0) | 26 (100.0) | 60 (100.0) | 102 (100.0) | |
| Do you have close friends? | | | | | |
| Yes, I do. | 15 (93.8) | 25 (96.2) | 60 (100.0) | 100 (98.0) | 0.201 |
| No, I do not. | 1 (6.3) | 1 (3.8) | 0 0 | 2 (2.0) | |
| Total | 16 (100.0) | 26 (100.0) | 60 (100.0) | 102 (100.0) | |

*n*(%).
*: $p < .05$. **: $p < .01$. ***: $p < .001$.

**Table 4.**
*Relationship between physical fitness test evaluation and school life.*

< 0.01) and played well with friends during play time (p < 0.001) (**Table 4**). Although it was not a significant difference, 80% of the children who answered "high" in the physical strength/athletic capability test said that school was fun. In addition, in the "I have good friends" item, there were almost no children answered it regardless of the high or low score of physical strength and physical capability test.

## 3.5 Relationship between physical strength, athletic capability evaluation test scores and lifestyle aspects

Children with high scores for physical strength and athletic capability clean up their surroundings and rooms more than children with low scores (p < 0.01) and many children answered that they would plan and study without saying ($p < 0.05$) (**Table 5**). Children with high scores for physical strength and athletic capability evaluation tests answered the following items: "stop when the time is decided in the middle of play", "decide what TV programs they want but do not watch constantly", "decide what they want to be in the future", and "there are things they want to do when they grow up." Although they answered many items, there was no significant difference. On the other hand, in the item of "staying at home alone" the "low" score was higher than "standard" and "high" scores.

### 3.6 The relationship between physical strength and athletic capability test scores and health aspect.

In the item "spending time well every day," it was found that many children with high scores responded "very cheerfully" ($p < 0.01$) (**Table 6**). In addition, the number of children who responded that their condition was worse was "frequently" or "sometimes occasionally" ($p < 0.05$), which had no significant difference. On the other hand, many of the children who scored "low" answered "frequently" or "sometimes" to be tired or to be feeling heavy.

| | | | | | |
|---|---|---|---|---|---|
| **I get up alone in the morning** | **7 (43.8)** | **13 (50.0)** | **29 (48.3)** | **49 (48.0)** | **0.923** |
| I stay at home alone | 13 (81.3) | 17 (65.4) | 41 (68.3) | 71 (69.6) | 0.525 |
| I clean up my surroundings and my room. | 2 (12.5) | 11 (42.3) | 34 (56.7) | 47 (46.1) | $0.006^{**}$ |
| I stop playing when the set time is over even during the play | 5 (31.3) | 13 (50.0) | 32 (53.3) | 50 (49.0) | 0.290 |
| I decide what TV programs I want to watch but do not watch constantly | 2 (12.5) | 8 (30.8) | 22 (36.7) | 32 (31.4) | 0.180 |
| I make plans and study even if not told | 1 (6.3) | 9 (34.6) | 27 (45.0) | 37 (36.3) | $0.016^{*}$ |
| I decide what I want to be in the future | 6 (37.5) | 11 (42.3) | 37 (61.7) | 54 (52.9) | 0.103 |
| There are things I want to try when I grow up | 8 (50.0) | 14 (53.8) | 34 (56.7) | 56 (54.9) | 0.886 |

*n*(%).
$^{*}$: $p < .05$. $^{**}$: $p < .01$.

**Table 5.**
*Relationship between physical fitness test scores and lifestyle aspects.*

| | Low | Standard | High | Total | Significance |
|---|---|---|---|---|---|
| I feel heavy and may be tired | | | | | |
| Frequently | 3 (25.0) | 1 (4.8) | 4 (8.2) | 8 (9.8) | 0.097 |
| Sometimes | 8 (66.7) | 8 (38.1) | 25 (51.0) | 41 (50.0) | |
| Not much | 0 0 | 8 (38.1) | 16 (32.7) | 24 (29.3) | |
| Never | 1 (8.3) | 4 (19.0) | 4 (8.2) | 9 (11.0) | |
| Total | 12 (100.0) | 21 (100.0) | 49 (100.0) | 82 (100.0) | |

| | Low | Standard | High | Total | Significance |
|---|---|---|---|---|---|
| I spend time well everyday | | | | | |
| Very well | 4 (33.3) | 7 (33.3) | 30 (61.2) | 41 (50.0) | 0.002** |
| Healthy person | 6 (50.0) | 14 (66.7) | 19 (38.8) | 39 (47.6) | |
| Not fine at all | 2 (16.7) | 0 0 | 0 0 | 2 (2.4) | |
| Total | 12 (100.0) | 21 (100.0) | 49 (100.0) | 82 (100.0) | |
| There's a time that I feel sick | | | | | |
| Often | 2 (16.7) | 1 (5.0) | 0 0 | 3 (3.7) | 0.037* |
| Sometimes | 7 (58.3) | 9 (45.0) | 20 (40.8) | 36 (44.4) | |
| Almost never | 3 (25.0) | 10 (50.0) | 29 (59.2) | 42 (51.9) | |
| Total | 12 (100.0) | 20 (100.0) | 49 (100.0) | 81 (100.0) | |

*n*(%).
*: $p < .05$. **: $p < .01$.

**Table 6.**
*The relationship between physical strength and athletic capability test scores and health aspect.*

## 3.7 The relationship between physical strength and athletic capability test and sleep time

Regardless of whether the physical strength and athletic capability test scores were high or low, the percentage of sleep time on weekdays was "more than 8 hours but less than 9 hours" (**Table 7**). On the other hand, during holidays, the percentage of children with high physical strength and athletic capability test scores of "high" was "more than 8 hours but less than 9 hours, but this was not a significant difference.

## 3.8 The relationship between physical strength and athletic capability test score and obesity

Although it was not a significant difference, there were many children whose physical strength and athletic capability test scores were "standard" and many of the

| | | Low | Standard | High | Total | Significance |
|---|---|---|---|---|---|---|
| Sleep time on weekdays | More than 6 hours but less than 7 hours | 0 0.0 | 2 (9.5) | 5 (10.2) | 7 (8.5) | 0.888 |
| | More than 7 hours but less than 8 hours | 3 (25.0) | 7 (33.3) | 15 (30.6) | 25 (30.5) | |
| | More than 8 hours but less than 9 hours | 7 (58.3) | 7 (33.3) | 18 (36.7) | 32 (39.0) | |
| | More than 9 hours but less than 10 hours | 2 (16.7) | 5 (23.8) | 10 (20.4) | 17 (20.7) | |
| | More than 10 hours | 0 0.0 | 0 0.0 | 1 (2.0) | 1 (1.2) | |
| | Total | 12 (100.0) | 21 (100.0) | 49 (100.0) | 82 (100.0) | |

| | | Low | Standard | High | Total | Significance |
|---|---|---|---|---|---|---|
| Sleep time on holidays | More than 6 hours but less than 7 hours | 0 0.0 | 1 (4.8) | 3 (6.5) | 4 (5.1) | 0.354 |
| | More than 7 hours but less than 8 hours | 1 (8.3) | 2 (9.5) | 7 (15.2) | 10 (12.7) | |
| | More than 8 hours but less than 9 hours | 8 (66.7) | 7 (33.3) | 17 (37.0) | 32 (40.5) | |
| | More than 9 hours but less than 10 hours | 0 0.0 | 8 (38.1) | 12 (26.1) | 20 (25.3) | |
| | More than 10 hours | 3 (25.0) | 3 (14.3) | 7 (15.2) | 13 (16.5) | |
| | Total | 12 (100.0) | 21 (100.0) | 46 (100.0) | 79 (100.0) | |

*n(%).*

**Table 7.**
*The relationship between physical fitness test and sleep time.*

| | Low | Standard | High | Total | Significance |
|---|---|---|---|---|---|
| Slender | 3 (18.8) | 4 (15.4) | 7 (11.7) | 14 (13.7) | 0.458 |
| Standard | 7 (43.8) | 17 (65.4) | 41 (68.3) | 65 (63.7) | |
| Obese | 6 (37.5) | 5 (19.2) | 12 (20.0) | 23 (22.5) | |
| Total | 16 (100.0) | 26 (100.0) | 60 (100.0) | 102 (100.0) | |

*N (%).*

**Table 8.**
*The relationship between physical fitness test score and obesity.*

children with "high" scores had "standard" body shapes (**Table 8**). However, about 20% of children who are slender and about 40% of those who are obese had "low" overall athletic capability test scores.

## 4. Discussion

In this study, for the purpose of clarifying the relationship between physical strength, athletic capability, school life, lifestyle, and health, we examined in detail the physical strength and athletic capability of both fifth-grade boys and girls such as their running power, jumping power, throwing power and endurance. As a result, the boys performed softball throwing repeatedly sideways, and a 20-m endurance runs while the girls performed a sit and reach test. In the physical strength test, the girls scored more than the boys. In addition, it was also suggested that children with high physical strength test scores were significantly higher in the aspects of school life, lifestyle, and health.

According to the 2016 national physical strength, athletic capability, and exercise habits survey results [9], in the fifth grade of elementary school, the average physical strength and athletic capability of boys was higher than that of girls in gripping strength, raising the upper body, repeated side jump, 20 m endurance run, standing long jump and softball throw. Moreover, the average value of girls was higher than that of boys in the sit and reach and in the 50 m run. However, the overall score was higher for girls than boys, and the results were similar to this study.

In addition, in this study, there was a difference between the minimum and maximum values in boys which was seen in the four events: repeated side jump, 20 m shuttle run, 50 m run, and standing long jump. In women's other events, the difference between the minimum and maximum values was small, but the difference was slight. From this, it is presumed that the physical strength level of boys who can exercise and those who cannot do is more polarized in boys than girls.

The tendency of the decline in the physical strength of children has been pointed out since the mid-1980s, and since the 2000s, the tendency of bipolarization has been taken up [10]. In relation to this, there were reports (Toyoshima [11, 12]) on the tendency of children's physical activity and the tendency to become bipolar in physical strength and athletic capabilities such as frequency of exercise for middle and high school students, long jump between 10 and 20 years old, shuttle run and ball throwing from elementary school to high school students, etc. There are extreme children who have a lot of physical activity and children who have little physical activity, or both children who have good physical strength and athletic capability and children who are inferior. In other words, it was recognized as a problem of "gap" [13].

In the lower grades of elementary school, students learn various basic movements such as walking, running, jumping, avoiding, turning, falling, floating, hanging, and climbing. And in the upper grades, it becomes possible to acquire the ability to combine various movements and develop the adjustment power, but there are gender differences and individual differences in physical strength/athletic capability and type of exercise. In addition, the difference is likely to increase with age, leading to bipolarization. It is important to experience various movements during this period called Golden Age. However, instead of capturing this time uniformly, I think it is important to give exercise guidance with due consideration of the developmental stages of elementary, middle, and upper grades.

According to the Niigata Physical Fitness and Life Survey [14], students with high scores and low scores with the new physical fitness test reported differences in living conditions. Atsuko [15] conducted a child QOL survey for parents and analyzed the relationship with physical activity, and reported that there were many steps for children with high health. Reizo [16] emphasizes the link between physical activity in childhood and the mental and physical health of the child. In this study as well, it was speculated that many children with high physical strength and athletic capability have good school life and good health and that physical strength and athletic capability affect their lifestyle.

The upper grades of elementary school are said to be the beginning of the time when the mind and body grow the most in a lifetime [17]. Therefore, in order to establish a healthy lifestyle, it is essential to form basic lifestyle, exercise, and physical activity habits during this period.

Hidetoshi [18] showed that the relationship between physique and motor skills in elementary school students showed that muscle power and instantaneous power of the upper limbs during throwing were affected by height and weight development, and increased Rohrer index with weight gain. It was suggested that it may be a factor to reduce the performance of exercise with physical movement. There were many children with physical strength/exercise capability test scores of "standard" and "high" for children whose body type was "standard." For this reason, further study is necessary on the relationship between body shape and athletic capability. In addition, this study is a cross-sectional study that was limited to a single academic year, so it is necessary to increase the number of regions and subjects and to conduct a longitudinal study in the future.

## 5. Conclusion

In this study, in order to clarify the relationship between children's physical strength, athletic capability, and school life and health, we collated and examined the results of the physical strength tests and questionnaire surveys of the said fifth graders. As a result, in the physical strength test, the boys performed softball throwing, repeated side jumps, and the 20 m shuttle run while the girls had a good performance with sit and reach test and there were more girls who scored higher than boys. In addition, it was confirmed that children with high scores for physical strength tests were found to be in good condition in terms of school life, health, and body shape.

The above suggests that physical strength and athletic capability are also related to children's school life and health and it was suggested that high physical strength had a positive impact on children's school life and health.

## Author details

Mijin Kim
Department of Children, Saitama Junshin Junior College, Japan

*Address all correspondence to: kim.m@sai-junshin.ac.jp

## References

[1] Ministry of Education, Culture, Sports, Science and Technology-Japan. 2018. Available from: http://www.mext.go.jp/b_menu/shingi/chukyo/chukyo0/gijiroku/attach/1344530.htm [Accessed: June 23, 2018].

[2] Ministry of Education, Culture, Sports, Science and Technology-Japan. About comprehensive measures for physical strength improvement of child (report). Available from: http://www.mext.go.jp/b_menu/shingi/chukyo/chukyo0/toushin/021001a.htm [Accessed: June 23, 2018]

[3] Central Education Council. About comprehensive measures for physical strength improvement of child (report). Teacher training. 2002;**31**:70-82

[4] Ministry of Education, Culture, Sports, Science and Technology-Japan. 2010 National Physical Strength・Exercise Ability, Exercise Habits Survey Report, Etc. Ministry of Education, Culture, Sports, Science and Technology; 2010. pp. 12-60

[5] Ministry of Education, Culture, Sports, Science and Technology-Japan. New Fitness Test - for a Significant Activity. Tokyo: Gyosei Publishing Company; 2000. pp. 1-54

[6] Ministry of Education, Culture, Sports, Science and Technology-Japan. Causes of reduced physical strength in children. 2014. Available from: http://www.mext.go.jp/b_menu/shingi/chukyo/chukyo0/gijiroku/attach/1344534.htm [Accessed: June 23, 2018]

[7] Keiko K, Akiko N, Atsushi Y. The relationship between children's physical strength/motor ability and lifestyle habits. To nurture the healthy mind and body of children from infancy to childhood. 2010. Available from: http://www.nps.ed.jp/nara-c/gakushi/kiyou/h22/2youji.pdf [Accessed: August 9, 2018]

[8] Noriko K, Mitsunori M, Miho K, Takashi T, Teruomi O. From the report of "study group on healthy child development through food". Pediatric Health Research. 2004;**63**:345-348

[9] Ministry of Education, Culture, Sports, Science and Technology-Japan. Survey result data such as 2016 national physical strength, athletic ability, exercise habits. 2016. Available from: http://www.mext.go.jp/sports/b_menu/toukei/kodomo/zencyo/1380529.htm [Accessed: August 20, 2019].

[10] Masaru K, Kayo T, Yoshinori K. Bipolarization of frequency of physical activity in childhood and adolescence. Japan Pediatric Society Magazine. 2004; **108**:625-634

[11] Kazufumi H, Kei T. Characteristics of boys and girls in the most superior and inferior groups on physical strength with progress of bipolarization of physical strength level. The growth development studies. 2008;**37**:57-67

[12] Hiroyuki T. Dynamics of sports exercise for children. Science of Physical Education. 2006;**56**(5):344-348

[13] Ikeda T, Aoyagi R. Relations between polarization in athletic capability and life environment factors in early childhood. Bulletin of Faculty of Human Sociology Fukuoka Prefectural University. 2016;**24**(2):23-39

[14] Niigata physical strength and life enforcement survey. 2018. Available from: https://www.pref.niigata.lg.jp/uploaded/attachment/40628.pdf [Accessed: December 3, 2018].

[15] Atsuko K. Physical activity and exercise intensity of young children. Science of physical education. 2008;**58**: 604-609

[16] Reizo B. What happens to children who do not exercise? Science of Physical Education. 2008;**58**:305-309

[17] Tokyo Minami-Tama nursery school, Hachioji-shi public health center, Machida-shi public health center. Healthy education booklet "Hop Step Jump" for elementary school 4th, 5th and 6th graders. 2007. Available from: http://www.fukushihoken.metro.tokyo.jp/minamitama/hakk [June 23, 2018].

[18] Hidetoshi M. A cross-sectional survey on the relationship between physique and athletic capability in elementary school students. Bulletin of Tokyo Future University. 2013;**6**:153-163

Chapter 2

# Accessible Resistance Movement Experiences for Elementary Students and Educators

*Alison Morag Murray, Pamela Murray and Kristy Howells*


## Abstract

What is meant by accessible resistance movement and why is the elementary education phase proposed as such a superb period in a child's life to gain competence and knowledge using resistance activity? This chapter presents a case and a means to do just that. The resistance program is called 'I Can Resist'. It is shared with accompanying pedagogical methods to scaffold learning and progress motor competence and biomotor fitness (agility that improves health through skill-related fitness). Interleaved through the progressions are ways to increase the self-management in how to participate in and create meaningful ways to improve targeted benefits. 'I Can Resist' is designed for novices to more experienced, participants and tutors alike. It was developed primarily for physical education supporting national curricular policy and implementation as regards knowledge and fitness outcomes. It was extended beyond the curriculum expectation in order to encourage greater use of the available affordances beyond the curriculum for lifelong health and well-being. Current findings are examined and insights offered. The 'I Can Resist' program is underpinned through research and theoretical application. It is showcased as interwoven with the means to develop agentic thinking and action. This ecological approach to and through resistance movement is contextually adaptable.


**Keywords:** developmentally appropriate, resistance, accessible, motor competent, pedagogy

## 1. Introduction

What does it mean to practice (educate) in a developmentally appropriate way? In essence, it means we go at the pace of the participant as they acquire the targeted and potential learning through meaningfully planned activities (scope) in a sensible order (sequence). There is a wee bit of nuanced room for emergent movement properties, beyond the planned foundational skills and accompanying competencies. Designed learning sequences need to be appropriate for the child's developmental level, rather than age or class level [1]. Within a practical learning domain, a developmentally appropriate scope and sequence will be informed by inclusive principles for children diverse in how they think, move and ultimately learn. Encouraging children to become more active for the sake of appreciation is an important objective for physical activity provision. Enjoyment has long since served as an antecedent of physical activity [2] and remains a subconstruct and strong indicator of intrinsic motivation [3]. To promote health relatable activity that interests and engages children during lessons in a developmental way is together challenging. Curricular time around meaningful physical activity is limited. Quality experiences, when meaningful and enjoyable, are likely to promote participation beyond mandated curriculum opportunities [4]. Often activity choice is curricular-driven and directed with carefully planned staged outcomes. Barriers and perceived barriers by children and youth need to be sensitively illuminated and addressed and related issues constructively resolved in efforts to increase the desire and the means to participate. Adolescence is acknowledged as a vulnerable phase. Growth slows and inactivity increases [5]. Youth can be very aware of how they look, and or how they feel they look in comparison to peers and or some external expectation. Body image satisfaction around perceptions and feelings around how one looks remains of seminal importance into early adulthood [6–8]. Unfortunately, body image is often low across the developmental stage [9]. Physiologically, children who are more active, tend to have lower levels of adipose tissue (body fat) as part of their body composition in contrast to more active peers [10]. This may also be an unfortunate, avoidable barrier as children try to engage in physical activity [11] where how they move is partly influenced by body composition. It is crucial to use only functional language. Communicating the function and purpose of body parts around body composition allows participants to learn and gain awareness in how to manage their bodies in non judgmental ways. Educating participants on the functional value of adipose tissue is a definitive starting point, and how to use empowering and task-oriented language is also a means to modelling ways to communicate around the body without triggering judgement of self and or others, performance and or body-wise. Furthermore, resistance problems can offer children and youth, diverse in needs and abilities and collective opportunities to learn through accessible yet resistance movements, sequences and challenges. Creative means to help children grow up respecting how they move and feeling comfortable enough to do in nurturing environments is crucial. Advising children on the need and benefits of all body composition components as well as the importance of their management of how they move makes for meaningful ways to keep the focus on the learning and away from spotlighting students as they enter the learning progressions. They too will present a broad range of needs and competencies and so program use needs to remain dynamic and responsive. It adopts more of a descriptive than prescriptive ethos whereby other ideas emerge as competence and confidence around such movement increases. Body image and mental health can be negatively impacted when social interactions are untoward [12]. I Can Resist is found to be effectively situated as just one part of a varied and contextually dynamic curriculum or complementary extracurricular affordance, rather than as a fixed point. Its components can also be applied through a wide range of topics, themes and curricular areas (subjects). It is but one means to advantage of limited space and engage children and youth in health-related experiential education. The accessibility is to ensure that educators varied in their competence, just as with our students, and have an equitable opportunity to include resistance movement as part of a holistic educational movement series.

In summary, a holistic, non-linear approach to the presented program is recommended. An explicit way to provide movement content knowledge and movement competence using individually preferred ways of being mobile create means by which participants take over ownership to use, adapt or progress beyond the first iteration is then possible. A functional approach can assist in accessibility and social acceptance, with the resistance band acting as an extension of the body and potential movement.

### 1.1 Not the 'F' word

What is it about fitness that turns thoughts, conversations and decisions? Skill-related fitness (SRF) consists of agility, balance, coordination, power, reaction time and speed [13]. Through SRF children are better able and equipped to access more ways to improve health and go on to explore other ways to enjoy a vigorous active life. With strategies to develop an independent understanding of exercise, in knowing what to do, how to do it, for how long and at what intensity, children can exercise informed judgements over making decisions important to living a healthy life [14]. These resistance challenges start from a simple to complex nature and remain engaging through creative use of FITT principles (frequency, intensity, time and type). Practically speaking, each component can be progressed through the incorporation of resistance work. Resistance training, generically defined as 'a form of periodic exercise whereby external weights provide progressive overload to skeletal muscles in order to make them stronger and often result in hypertrophy' [15], p. 208), is popular across society and used for a variety of purposes inclusive of strength training for recreation, for health and rehabilitation and for sports performance. In parallel with a lifelong approach to health and well-being denoted through physical educational guidelines across the globe [16, 17], the UK presents guidelines that adopt a lifelong approach through physical activity participation [18]. Through policy, physical activity is encouraged across the day from as early as infancy, from such a thirty-minute distributed time allotment, toddlers extend at least three hours daily in a variety of distributed physically active time. Pre-schoolers are then encouraged to increase the effort exerted within that time. Children of school age ought to be physically active for at least 60 minutes daily. Again, variety is encouraged and importantly, activities that develop movement skills, muscular fitness and bone strength [19] are advocated. The UK Chief Medical Officers emphasise the importance of strengthening activities in childhood. Furthermore, activities that provide periods of high-intensity interval exercise provide beneficial effect to fitness, body weight and insulin resistance (2019; 8). Children across elementary health-related require a daily average of 60 minutes of moderate-to-vigorous activity. Physical education is acknowledged as part of this, alongside after-school activity [18, 20]. How much is too much and hard is too hard? Children in most deprived areas of England are found as most obese in relation to peers living elsewhere [21]. Surely, we can position a socially just exciting affordance for children and adolescents regardless of home address and zip code? Worldwide adolescents are trending as inactive and therefore not meeting guidelines [22]. This means moving beyond traditional activities and/or traditional ways to access appear salient ways to arouse interest and increase engagement.

'I Can Resist' provides a range of body resistance challenges across a varied series of ways to try these ahead of explicit implementation of choices to use the bands. Of itself, this also provides a super field formative assessment to inform the tutor of how the participant manages their body and manages their body when movement skills are presented, modelled and explained, and then made into more complex sets and sequences and implemented into other activity and game forms. Intensity-wise, it is also vital we provide practical means for children to develop their awareness of what effort means and how their bodies respond to such exertion. A student-directed approach reflects the ecological nature underpinning the program and its holistic implementation. *'I can talk and practice'*—light, *'I can talk and engage but am out of breath'*—medium, *'I need to do the exercises first and then rest and talk'*—high intensities can be gently introduced, modelled and experienced within programmed time. Pedagogically, effort, together with actual challenges, can be experienced and increased through solo, peer and group endeavours.

### 1.2 F-word summary

For a series of timeproof reasons, many students are turned off by fitness, and sadly statutory linear outcome expectations have further impoverished its image. Let us clean up and embrace functional language as we live this F word!

### 1.3 Physical activity, motor competency through physical education

From a motoric standpoint, Gabbard [23] illustrates the significant role of motor competence through life span. Physical education programmes should provide concentrated instruction in basic movement skills needed to enjoy a variety of skills [24]. Fundamental skills need to be acquired ahead of advanced and for that reason, expectations to experience and master these through elementary physical education are depicted [25, 26] as policy enactment exemplars of the UNESCO Charter of Physical Education and Sport (1978). Freedoms to 'develop physical, intellectual and moral powers' when facilitated through developmentally relevant means within the respective educational system, open opportunities beyond these. As an 'essential element of education and culture', physical education (and sport) has been prioritised as an 'essential element of lifelong education' ([17]; Article 2.1).

In England, the nominal expectations for elementary-aged children are two hours of physical education a week [25]. This length of time is acknowledged as insufficient to appropriate adequate physical education active learning time for children to become proficient in movement skills [1]. Students should be actively moving 50–80% of this time [27]. There are pupils within the national primary curriculum temporal span who lack competency in movement proficiency [28]. This is all the more complex when emergent movement is part of the joy of the experience. Moves, unplanned and unanticipated, are often part of an exciting movement experience. If then, motor skill competence promotes participation [29], we do need to have contemplated how we balance planned and emergent skill acquisition and implementation. Keeping that ambiguity is part of a wider embodiment of the complexity of physically educating [30]. Such complexity thinking can serve as a principle to further opening access to enjoyable physical activity.

In England, some children are found to be inactive from as young as five years of age [31]. Children participating in the United States can expect a minimum of 150 minutes weekly at the primary level, increasing to 225 minutes through secondary levels [26]. The U.S. Department of Health and Human Services recommend that students engage in more than 50% of class time at moderate-to-vigorous activity levels [32]. Regular physical activity promotes a variety of physical and mental health benefits yet a majority of children have systematically struggled to meet guidelines [33, 34]. Intensity levels within these expectations become even more problematic to attain let alone measure when children are less motor competent. Pupils without proficiency in movement skills have exhibited lower levels of physical activity participation than their peers during school break times [35, 36]. Barriers (such as screen time) and facilitators (such as physical education and home-based activity) to physical activity are varied [37]. Nonparticipation in physical activity is attributed to equal complexity and decisive action and has been prominent through holistic approaches to increase physical activity within physical education [38]. Cognitive functioning is accepted as pivotal for the successful engagement in health-related elements of developing health [39]. Further compromise was created by the educational closures as a result of the COVID-19 pandemic reductions in physical fitness, together with increases in mental distress [40].

Physical education programmes should provide concentrated instruction in basic movement skills needed to develop a variety of skills [24]. As determined through its philosophical underpinning and attributed value, it will seek to educate through determined criteria to attain and surpass curricular expectations for all children of all abilities and needs. The notion of attaining fitness-specific outcomes with all children, diverse in needs, is inherently challenging [41]. Some children do not enjoy the subject. Some children do so yet may be less enthusiastic regarding fitness-specific activities. Others may thrive across the settings regardless of pedagogies or topics. Explicit strategies to support child enjoyment are required [42]. The environment offers potential interest for children. In schools where space beyond the school building is a premium, the use of the playground can exploit limited areas and offer opportunities to develop motor skills, providing opportunities for action as determined by the environmental stimulus [43]. When physical education is constrained through time and space, such additional affordance can extend learning beyond the physical education experience. Greater creativity during the multiple considerations for children regarding their health through physical education widens the scope of plausible solutions. Health-related fitness, namely flexibility and coordination, cardiovascular endurance, muscular strength and endurance, with metabolic components [44], is accessible and improved as motor competence improves. Motor competence, motor ability and coordination as practised through fundamental motor skills [45] are determined essential for the development of a healthy and active lifestyle [46]. Motor competence has been found to be a significant predictor of HRF through locomotor skills and for boys using locomotor and manipulative skills [46]. Globally, such essential skills are incorporated into curricular elementary education.

### 1.4 Summary

If we wish children to get more excited about how they move, we need to facilitate exciting movement opportunities. We need to listen to our adolescents even more so that they get the chance to do more of what they enjoy in and around the school setting. That way they will become part of the solution in creating other opportunities in the wider community. Physical education has effectively used a part of a wider approach to educate and engage children and adolescents. Pedagogy—how we teach this Pedagogy and the way we enact it communicate so much to students as regards who we are and who we think they are. A social constructivist approach to knowledge acquisition would place emphasis on the active role of the learner in constructing respective knowledge with appropriate and explicit guidance and scaffolding form an informed entity; traditionally a teacher [47]. Personal and social perspectives toward the creation of knowledge can each play an important role in pupil education [48].

How we facilitate learning is as important as the knowledge, competencies and concepts explored themselves. The role of the program, in part, is to improve awareness and functionality so that participants become more able and apt to explore other activities and pursuits following completion of both the scaffolded body movement management learning sequence and the commitment resistance band program. From a participant's perspective, interests and preferences will vary greatly across family and community contexts and so the way the information is shared and how it is experienced during and around the curriculum wants to sound and feel exciting. Accessing physical activity relies upon being motor competent and cognizant. The I Can Resist program goes through all basics in what, how and where and we move practical means using, managing their bodies as they move through different planes and directions in closed to more open environments, without and then using manipulatives. Its pedagogical element ensures that an understanding of why we do so is developed through the experience. The development of self-awareness enables the collective body to become more aware of one another. Being and keeping a conscious awareness of the diversity across the class/group enables us pragmatically to open our awareness in non-judgmental ways [49] and model that to our participants. As educators, how we support learning through our language, as expressed through what and we say what we communicate, is collectively as important as what we actually do. Such practice sits companionably beside a curriculum as well as within it. Once 'bodies' have experienced how to move in differing directions, at different levels and using varied points of contact (e.g. one wheelset and two feet, for example, equate one to two points of contact) through varied movement concepts (e.g. explored alone, shared with a partner, mirroring or following a partner, at a very slow tempo and so on), participants are invited to participate in other tasks and challenges and resistance-based games drawing from (and thereby learning) the I Can Resist movement bank (**Tables 1** and **2**). The I Can Resist introductory progression spiral prepares the participant for a series of traditional resistance exercises, each and all of which can be more meaningfully implemented through a progression spiral approach. Movement challenges can be created by tutors and students, games can be modified to incorporate lower, core and upper resistance tasks, all of which proffer benefits without or with the added resistance band. Once participants can manage their bodies through resistance with coordinated control, they can attend to the added cognitive and physical challenge of doing so with the resistance band [50]. To create an accessible and enjoyable experience series, all children should have the appropriate time needed to gain self-body management through resistance exercises before progressing to an added piece of equipment. Participants become accustomed to an educational progression spiral (viz. learning driven such as through skill-task-challenge-game application). However, if you choose to implement the program to reflect your philosophies and desired to learn, avoid slipping into a fitness set. It always ends with the cessation of something. Keeping it educationally accessible is an authentic attempt to do just that. You may have other helpful means. Use sporadically as part of a spiral wider curriculum/program so that the experience stays meaningful. You can return to and progress it as when it supports your learning and resistance experience intentions. A simple A-B-C approach works well and can be conflated to work toward goals and intentions.

a. A light dynamic movement warm-up and educational elicitation to the experience (skill-activity-game-based challenges to open the inquiry and the interest to learn more).

DOI: http://dx.doi.org/10.5772/intechopen.110179

| | | |
|---|---|---|
| #1. Squats (quadriceps and hamstrings) | 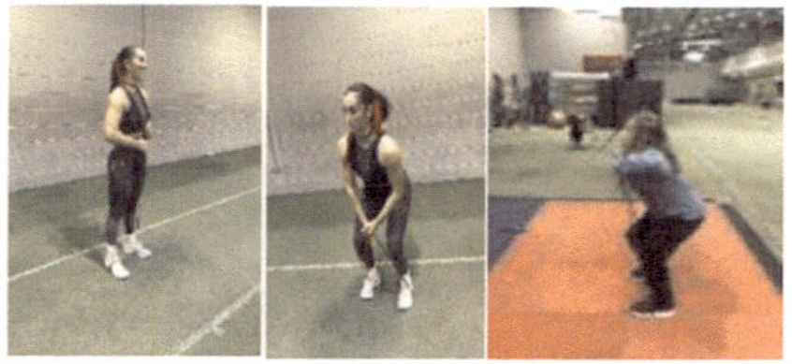 | Begin in a standing position and feet shoulder-width apart. With your hands in front begin to squat down (as if to sit in and get out of a chair). Squat down until you feel tightness in your thighs. Again, keep your hands in the front and stand back straight. |
| #2. Hamstring (and gluteus maximus) resistance curl and extensions | 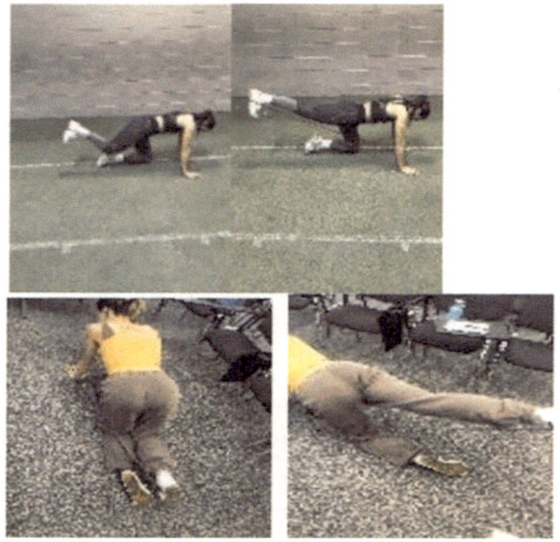 | Begin face down using four point contact stable position. Anchor band under hands and set around foot (like a stirrup). Drive one leg back and hold. |
| #?. Floor star shapes. Floor 4-point contact points (hand-hand-foot-foot**) position Star positions can incorporate L, C, and U areas. | 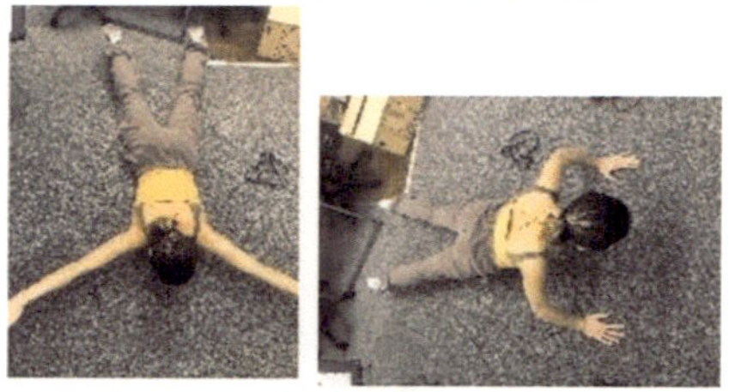 | Face down extended body position Feet and hands can contact (4 points) or be raised off the ground. Can add resistance band over shoulders, anchoring band at each hand contact over shoulders. |

| | | |
|---|---|---|
| #3. Reverse lunge/*forward lunge (*only when comfortable)/Side lunge<br>Formative assessment<br>A cross (flag) shape- forwards, backwards and to the sides provide a very accessible formative assessment of stability.<br>Participants will need control in these directions and changing levels before they add complexity (such as skill combinations and or added resistance).<br>Participants to show and tell as in try the set and explain how it is done and why to provide a formative point of understanding and competence. | 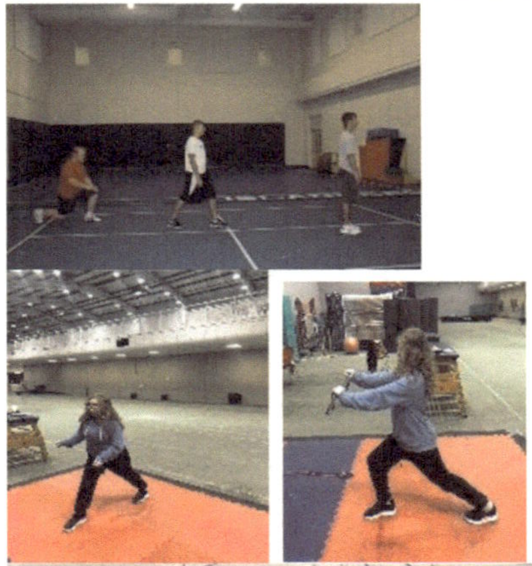 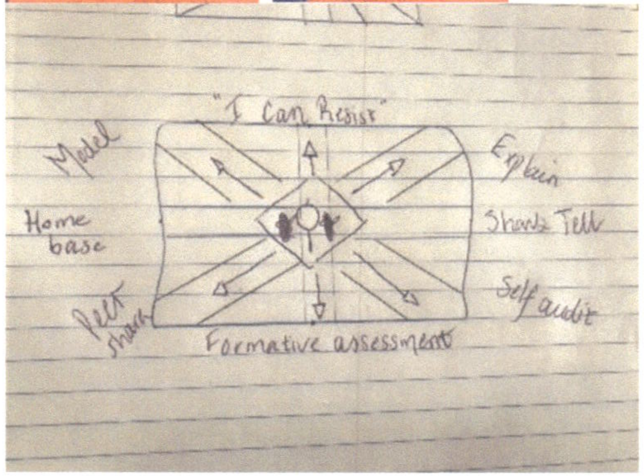  | Anchor the band at the level of the ground. Standing, hook your foot around the band and take the leg backwards. Bend the knees into a lunge position, keep knee behind the foot and hold for one second. Slowly return to starting position, Both legs.<br>For formative assessment- competence and understanding. Show the British union flag as a movement guide to show the directions, show and explain forwards, backwards straight and diagonals. Use and adapt to appropriate access: A) With body only, and hands-free, b) holding the band in front and then c) using the band to increase the difficulty of the lunge. Start and return to home base each time. |

DOI: http://dx.doi.org/10.5772/intechopen.110179

| | | |
|---|---|---|
| #4. Single-leg and double-squat thrust repeats (quadriceps and gluteus maximus) | 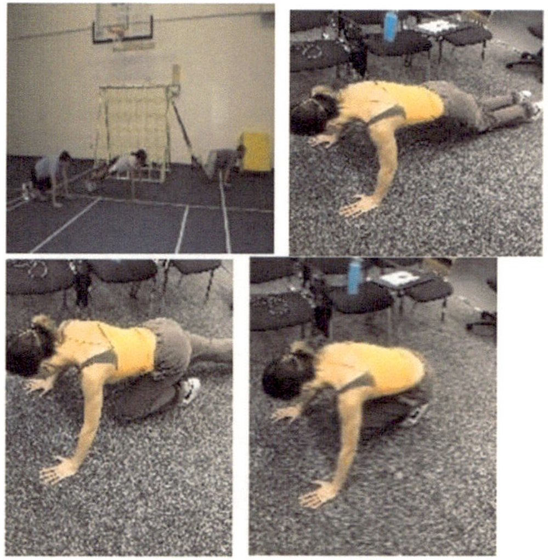 | In push-ups/plank position, bring one of your legs forward, so as to touch your knee to the chest and bring it back. Repeat this with the opposite leg. Try legs at the same time for a double squat thrust. |
| #5. Heel Raise (gastrocnemius) | 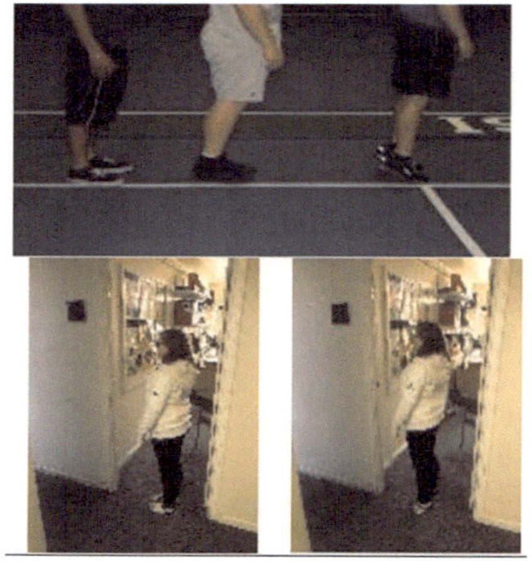 | Stand with toes on the raised platform and heels on the ground. Lift your heels keeping the toes on the balance bar until you feel the tension in your calf muscles. Return back to starting position. |

| | | |
|---|---|---|
| #6. Seated/standing tibial toe raise | 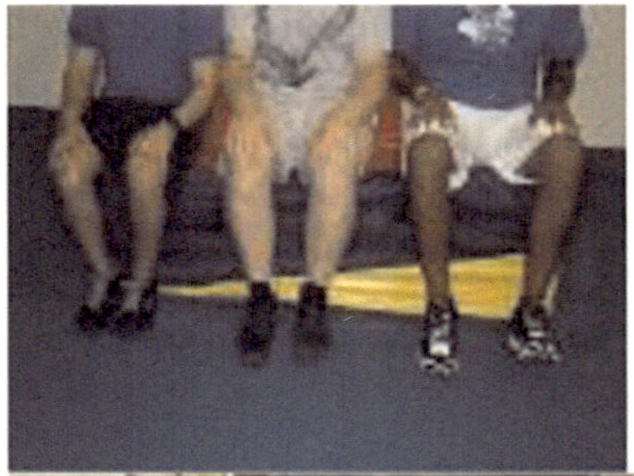 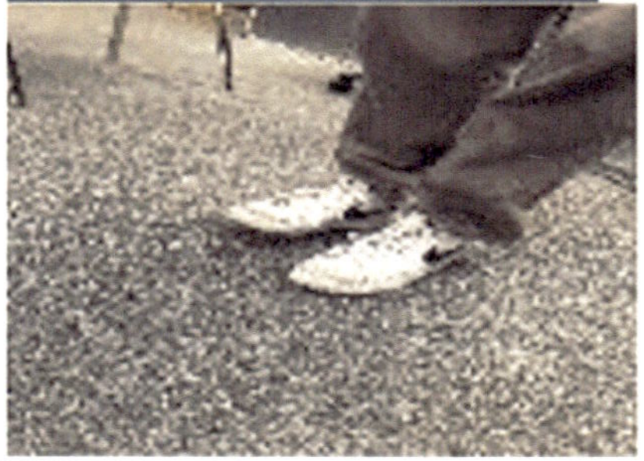 | In a seated position, bent legs assume a 90-degree angle with feet knees and hips parallel to shoulders. Raise toes of both feet while keeping the heel on the ground (dorsiflexion). For standing toe raise, feet in parallel position, shoulder-width apart. |
| #7. Adapted versions of 1–6 to suit; engage and inspire learner ** | Creative combos? Peer led | Peer/group ideas and creations. |

DOI: http://dx.doi.org/10.5772/intechopen.110179

| | | |
|---|---|---|
| #8. Curl up (rectus abdominus) | 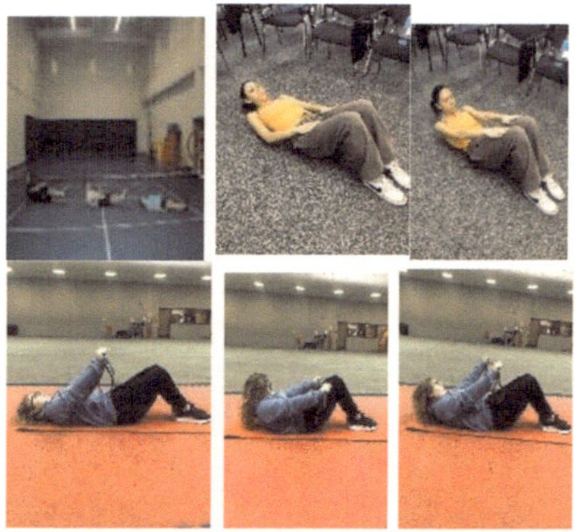 | Assume a lying position with arms parallel to the body. Hands remain in contact with the ground bring your chin toward your chest by lifting your shoulders and then return to the start position. Bend legs at the knee. |
| #9. V – Sit (rectus and transverse abdominus) | 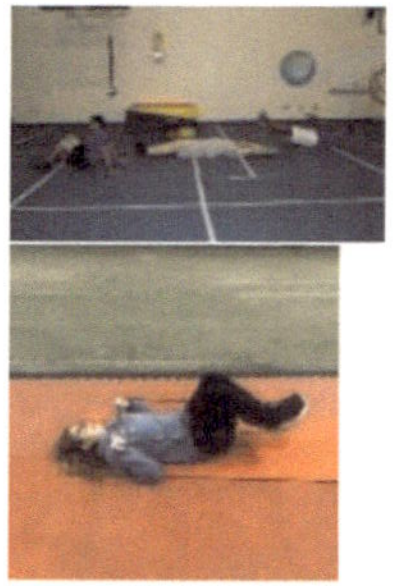 | Assume a sitting position and lean back to take weight on your hands (hands facing forward). Raise feet off ground and bring knees into the chest. With feet off ground extend your legs forward. Repeat action. |
| #10. Plank<br>Side plank (oblique abdominal) | 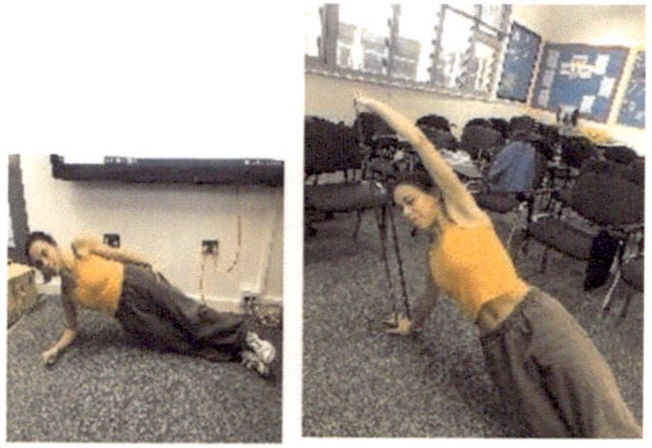 | Lower to floor position and extend into a side plank. Raise hips and knees off the floor. Keep head and spine neutral (keep tension through core).<br>Add resistance by raising top arm and/or with band. |

| | | |
|---|---|---|
| #11. Seated row (back and forearms) | 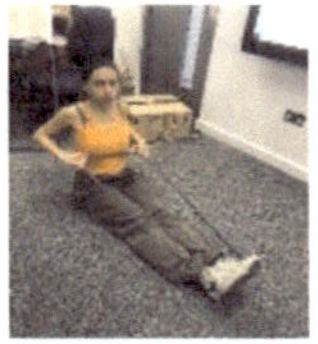 | In seated position, with back straight and chest open, anchor the band around both feet (like stirrups). Pull the band toward abdomen and squeeze shoulder blades together. Keep back straight across; pull elbows back, staying close to sides, controlled release and repeat. |
| #12. Back extension (erector spinae and gluteus) | 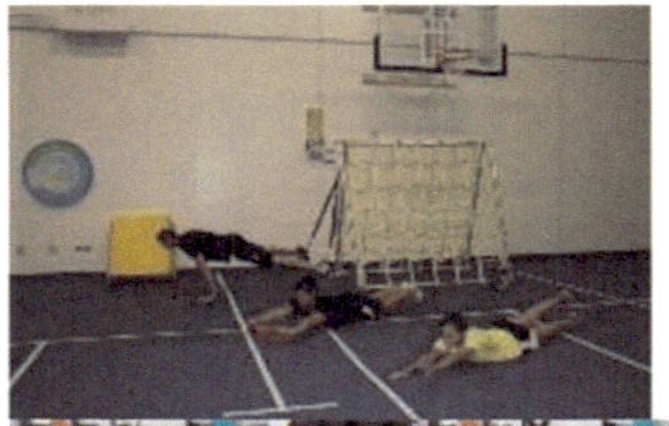 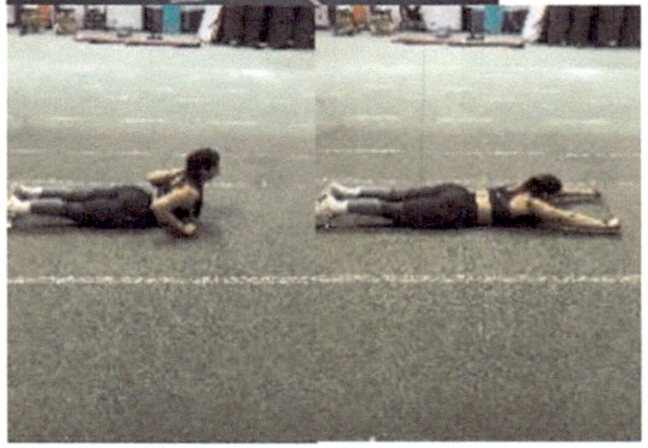 | Lie on stomach. Hold resistance band in hands and stretch it. Raise both hands and legs at the same time. Return back to start position and repeat action. |
| #13. Standing shoulder press | 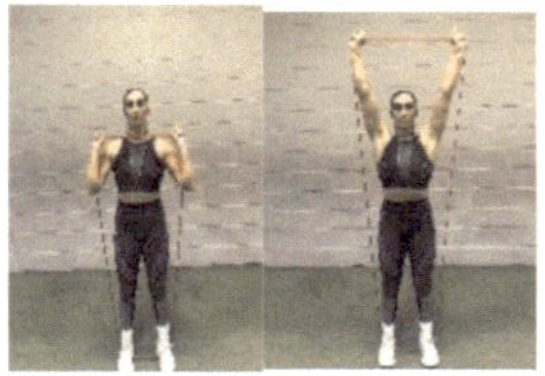 | Anchor band under feet and drive arms straight up. Keep core engaged. |

DOI: http://dx.doi.org/10.5772/intechopen.110179

| | | |
|---|---|---|
| #14. Mini push up (chest; pectoralis, with upper body and core) to plank and back to push up position repeats.<br>Resistance push ups—only if the position is stable | 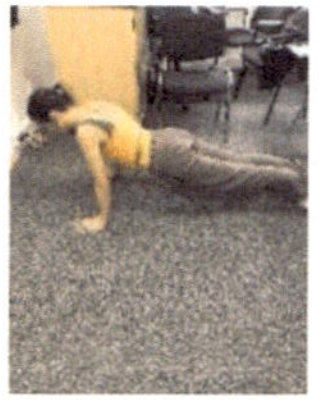 | Push-up position; (focus effort to avoid sagging banana and high bridge shapes). Press to change position from hands to forearms and back.<br>Anchor band under hands, extend over shoulders and move into a plank position, bend arms to lower chest and keep body tension. Take out slack of band and try to push upwards. |
| #15. Upright row (shoulders, upper back, delts and traps) | 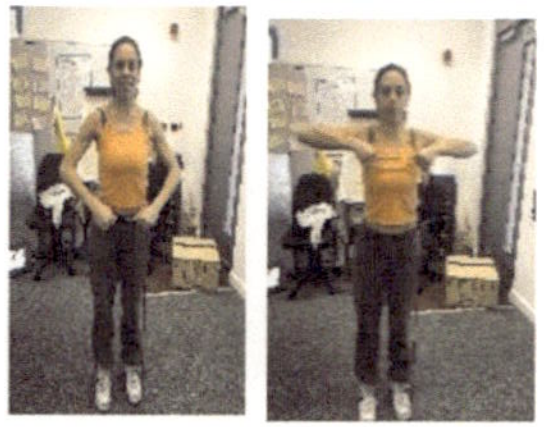 | Stand, feet shoulder-width apart, stand on band to anchor it, then hold with both hands to pull the band up toward chin level. Lead with elbows, pause at top, slow release and repeat. |
| #16. Adapted versions of 8–16 to suit; engage and inspire learner | Creative combos? Peer-led | Peer/group ideas and creations |
| #17. Latissimus dorsi pull down | 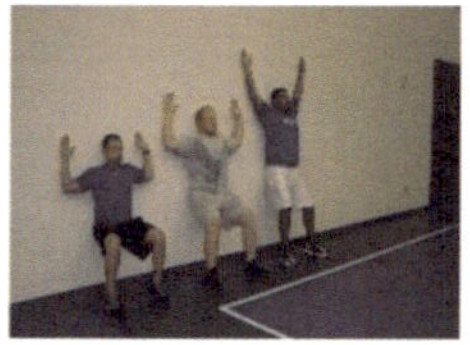 | Assume wall squat position. Raise arms to stick-up position with arms pressed against wall and elbows parallel to shoulder level. Maintaining contact with wall, pull arms down to shoulder level. Return to start position and repeat action.<br>Can add band. Standing, add resistance by pulling both ends of the band extended above the head. Lower arms in front chest level and repeat. |

| | | |
|---|---|---|
| #18. Deltoids (and trapezius) lateral raise | 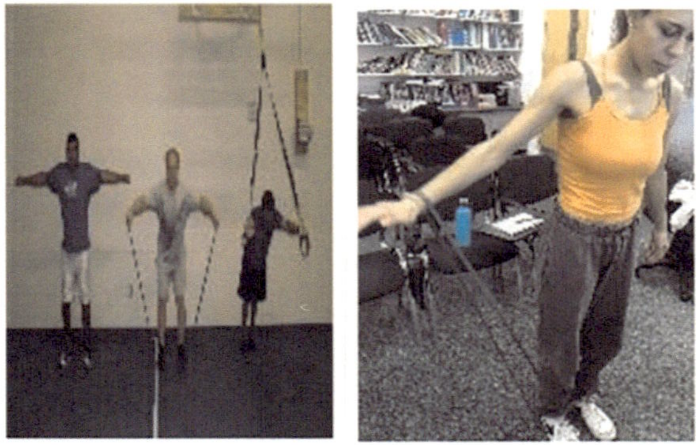 | In standing position, raise arms from extended position parallel to body up to shoulder level and return to the start position.<br>Repeat action. |
| #19. Biceps curl | 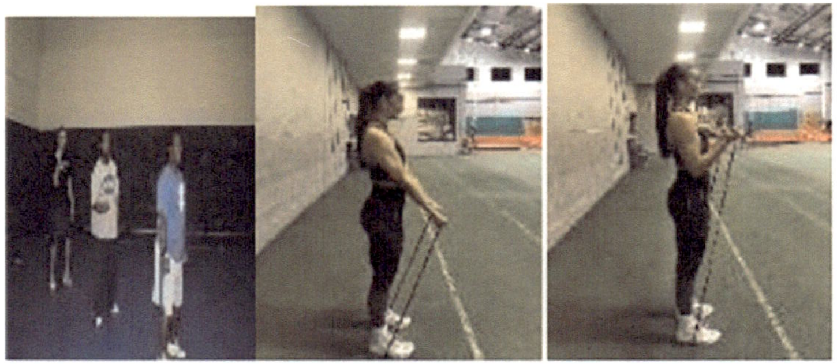 | Stand straight with knee slightly bent. Bend arm at elbow to bring hand toward shoulder. Return to the start position and repeat action. |
| #20. Triceps extension | 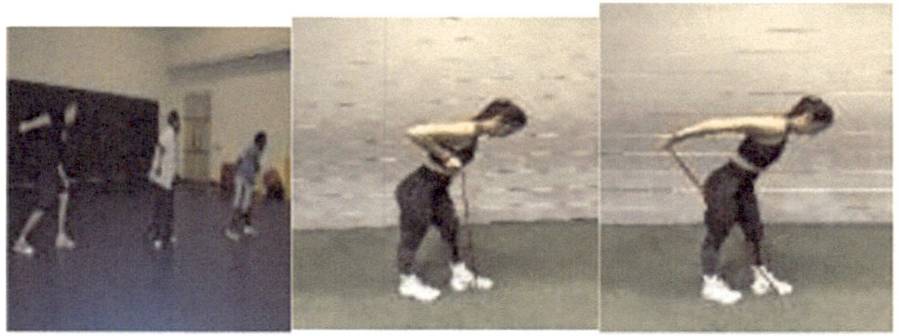 | Anchor the resistance band under the foot on the opposite side (diagonal) to extending arm. Lean forwards, and with a high elbow parallel to the body, try to straighten and extend arm back. Hold then gently release and repeat. |

| | | |
|---|---|---|
| #21. Combinations of 2–3 exercises sequentially connected (supersets) | L,C,U combinations | Peer/group led |
| #22. Adapted versions of 17–21 to suit; engage and inspire learner | Creative combos? Peer led | Peer/group ideas and creations |

*N.B. accessibility: #seven, 16 and 22 invites and encourage all pupils and tutors to use these creatively to ensure all children can access and improve their motor competence and confidence as their health and skill-related fitness improve. Choices. Make your own pics for your own class/group relatable series.*

**Table 1.**
*Accessible resistance movement bank-basic exercise name, primary muscle engaged (only), description and image for lower (L), core (C) and upper body (U) development, adapt to the participant's preferred mode of mobility.*

| |
|---|
| #1. Squats (quadriceps and hamstrings) |
| #2. Hamstring (and gluteus maximus) resistance curl and extensions |
| #? Floor star shapes. Floor 4-point contact points (hand-hand-foot-foot**) position |
| #3. Reverse lunge/*forward lunge (*only if comfortable), England flag lunge challenge |
| #4. Single-leg and double squat thrust repeats (quadriceps and gluteus maximus) |
| #5. Heel raise (gastrocnemius) |
| #6. Seated/standing tibial toe raise |
| #7. Adapted versions of 1–6 to suit, engage and inspire learners ** |
| #8. Curl up (rectus abdominus) |
| #9. V–Sit (rectus and transverse abdominus) |
| #10. Plank (rectus abdominis, obliques, and transverse abdominis) and side plank (oblique abdominal) |
| #11. Seated row (back and forearms) |
| #12. Back extension (erector spinae and gluteus) |
| #13. Standing shoulder press |
| #14. Mini push up (chest; pectoralis, with upper body and core) to plank and back to push-up position repeats,<br>Resistance band Push ups |
| #15. Upright row (shoulders, upper back; delts and traps) |
| #16. Adapted versions of 8–16 to suit; engage and inspire learner |
| #17. Latissimus dorsi pull down |
| #18. Deltoids (and trapezius) Lateral raise |
| #19. Biceps curl |
| #20. Triceps extension |
| #21. Combinations of 2–3 exercises sequentially connected |
| #22. Adapted versions of 17–21 to suit, engage and inspire learner |

**Table 2.**
*Summary.*

b. The experience sequence (through whichever medium fits context and informs and inspires the group). This, following the first explicit progression spiral, is then ready for adaptations and or to be swapped out by self/group/class-created and generated iterations.

c. Plenary to revisit any points to progress further, to respond to movement questions and acknowledge meaningful movement responses from the participants (with a light cool down), again as interests the group and constructively completes the engagement.

Developmentally appropriate rest (and quality water breaks) is and remains student-determined and led. Use holistic means to sensibly and safely manage the participation experience time. Active rest through participation for light to moderate intensity participation use water break walking reflections between more intense bouts. Use a holistic approach to intensity, for example, perceived intensity guide: Child initiated is important to model and facilitate that ownership toward self-awareness and agency—'I can talk and practice'—light, 'I can talk and engage but am out of breath'—medium, 'I need to do the exercises first and then actively rest, for example, walk and talk'—high intensity). Always adapt to engage and inspire every learner. Know and accommodate participant constraints and expectations ahead of time [51]. Work alongside participants and have them inform/show you what works for them. Encourage peer opportunity and creative use of concepts to engage children through cooperative and competitively cooperative means to experience the challenges. Competition (against self and others) can be interpreted in ways meaningful to the respective group at the respective time in the respective context across the curriculum/learning journey. For example, the program can be explicitly used for challenges and ways such as using effective communication and peer modelling to create, present and even compete in dynamic resistance band routines set to student-chosen instrumental music. It can also be reduced implicitly (following skill acquisition and competence attainment) through modified adventures, games and pursuits.

## 2. Summary

The emergent nature surfaces following explicit scaffolding of the basics through the I Can resist progression spiral which is holistically designed to develop both movement and self-management competence through self and socially interactive opportunities. Participant ownership then creates further affordances to engage in meaningful resistance movement activities following explicit modelling and explanation of the basics. This simply provides an equitable entry point for all and then is used and imagined on their terms.

## 3. Current findings exploring resistance movement activities in and around the curriculum

Strength-related activities improve daily function and self-esteem children varied in functional gross motor proficiency [52]. In regards to biomotor abilities (strength, endurance, speed, flexibility and coordination), children and youth made significant improvements across aerobic endurance, strength endurance, flexibility and body composition (as indirectly measured through waist-to-height ratio) when implementing the program twice weekly as is and once weekly through an educational games version as measured using the FITNESSGRAM [53]. **Tables 3–7** depict the number of participants across the control and three groups using the program through differing pedagogies. All four groups participated in daily physical education classes across the academic year and participated in the pre- and post-experimental implementation. Each enumerated grouping (1–4) included several classes from both one elementary and one secondary school setting. Groups 2, 3 and 4 all experienced significant improvements in their biomotor fitness components. Those from the control experienced a significant reduction. Results depict between participant effects. Means are displayed to denote any changes between pre- and post-daily physical education curricular programmes, three of which were dedicated to the biomotor-focused resistance program. Following the attainment of institutional and school district ethical permissions, elementary and middle schools volunteered to participate. The eight schools were randomly assigned to training (three cohorts of 250; n = 750) as implemented using a variety of more direct to less direct teaching styled choices and one cohort as control (N = 250). All groups participated in daily PE (60 minutes). Those in the control group participated in the respective school curriculum and dedicated two days weekly to fitness-related activity. Those in the training groups participated in the resistance exercise program across two (out of five) lessons in their curriculum. All schools provided games-focused activities across the remainder days (court and field games). The main outcomes found significant improvement in biomotor competencies (as measured through the FITNESSGRAM). Cohorts across a series of state elementary and secondary schools participated through control and three pedagogical iterations of the resistance program to explore tutor and participant preference. The direct teaching group (n = 201) demonstrated significantly improved scores across fitness biomotor competencies measured ($z = -5.763$, $p < 0.001$). Those in the inquiry-based cohort (n = 174) significantly improved their fitness ($z = -4.439$, $p < 0.001$). Pupils within the combined group of resistance as delivered through

| Treatment | Fitness | Mean | Std. error |
|---|---|---|---|
| Control | 1 | 101.815 | 4.087 |
| | 2 | 85.444 | 4.312 |
| Direct | 1 | 84.404 | 3.669 |
| | 2 | 99.115 | 3.871 |
| Inquiry | 1 | 102.960 | 3.943 |
| | 2 | 114.920 | 4.160 |
| Inquiry-direct | 1 | 102.556 | 4.477 |
| | 2 | 107.378 | 4.723 |

**Table 3.**
*Mean changes from pre (1) to post (2) measurement across four groups (elementary and secondary student combinations) in the treatment of biomotor fitness components through three differing pedagogical iterations implementing the same content program content, competencies and knowledge.*

| Self-management | Pre | Post | Change |
|---|---|---|---|
| Mean | 2.42 | 2.59 | 0.18 |
| Number of items measured in responses (of participants present) | 6253 | 6226 | 27 |

**Table 4.**
*Mean score and change across questions around self-management (metacognition) of physical activity.*

| | Number of responses | % of responses |
|---|---|---|
| That stayed the same | 4441 | 72% |
| That increased | 1388 | 22% |
| That decreased | 380 | 6% |

**Table 5.**
*Score changes between the pre- and post-self-management measurement.*

| | Pre | Post | Change |
|---|---|---|---|
| Mean | 3.75 | 3.88 | 0.13 |
| Number of items measured by responses (of participants present) | 4876 | 4879 | 3 |

**Table 6.**
*Motivation pre and post change.*

| Motivation | Number of responses | % of responses |
|---|---|---|
| That stayed the same | 2568 | 53% |
| That increased | 1367 | 28% |
| That decreased | 905 | 19% |

**Table 7.**
*Mean score and change in score, all motivation questions combined.*

direct–indirect combination teaching method (n = 135) demonstrated significant improvements across the collective fitness regimen ($z = -6.902$, $p < 0.001$). Pupils in the control group (n = 162) did not improve their fitness. This reduced significantly ($z = -3.675$, $p < 0.001$) (**Table 3**).

Following this inquiry, it became imperative to explore how to maximise physical education (PE) provision for settings where the academic subject was provided limited time (twice weekly). Therefore, if PE allocated time could not encompass adequate time to improve biomotor fitness, it could arguably be used to prepare children and to motivate them to learn how to use such skills in ways they found enjoyable in and beyond PE. This function was integrated into the next research series, linking curricular PE to recess physical activity. Institutional and local authority ethical permissions were sought and attained for this quasi-experimental study. Participating schools in South England incorporated explicit teaching to participating children and youth on how to exercise and perform the moves safely and effectively. Basic skills were introduced, explained and modelled during PE through teacher-led sequences. Explicit attention was provided to the explicit training of educators and interested (student) participants for recess time peer-initiated participation following the introduction and practice of the skills in PE time. Both motivations to join in and continue this beyond class time, together with knowledge of how to execute and regulate self-participation significantly improved as measured through developmentally appropriate intrinsic motivation and metacognitive awareness inventories [3, 54]. Participants significantly improved declarative, procedural and contextual knowledge around the skills and competencies acquired in PE and then transferred to extracurricular peer-led physical activity following a five-month intervention ($x = 0.400$, $n = 6226$, $p < 0.001$). Awareness of how to use resources beyond the PE setting learning was significantly higher in the post-condition compared to the pre-condition ($z = -22.86$, $r = -0.29$, $p < 0.001$). Unlike that of the directed PE time, when scaffolded in a way that opened participant choice of how and when the resistance challenges were used, motivation to participate during lunchtime, with peer invitation and support increased. In all participants there was a larger number whose score increased (mean $\pm$ s.e. = 195 $\pm$ 8.37) than decreased (129 $\pm$ 3.82) although the majority of scores stayed the same (367 $\pm$ 7.41).

Metacognition was measured. Findings show that the level of participant metacognitive awareness, with regard to their use of the playground markings, increased from the beginning to the end of the study and that this difference was statistically significant ($x = 0.400$, $n = 6226$, $p < 0.001$) [55]. Scores were significantly higher post-treatment compared to pre-treatment in both function groups although the effect size was larger for regulation of cognition (Wilcoxon Signed Rank test: $z = -13.78$, $r = -0.25$, $p < 0.001$) than it was for knowledge of cognition ($z = -18.26$, $r = -0.33$, $p < 0.001$). Consistent with this, the regulation cognition group of questions were associated with a substantially larger number and proportion of increases in response score from pre- to post-treatment than were the knowledge of cognition question. The mean knowledge of cognition scores were higher than the mean regulation of cognition scores both pre- (Knowledge: 2.60' Regulation: 2.23) and post (Knowledge: 2.73; Regulation: 2.46) treatment but the change in score was greater for regulation of cognition (Regulation +0.22; Knowledge: +0.13) (**Tables 4** and **5**).

Motivation to participate using a variety of moves in student-directed ways during lunch was appraised via the motivation scores. These scores were significantly higher in the post-condition compared to the pre-condition and when the questions were considered separately, scores were significantly higher post-treatment compared to pre-treatment in five out of the seven questions. In all cases, there was a larger number of students whose score increased (mean $\pm$ s.e. = 195 $\pm$ 8.37) than decreased (129 $\pm$ 3.82) although the majority of scores stayed the same (367 $\pm$ 7.41). (**Tables 6** and **7**). Unsurprisingly opportunities to share some ownership of how such a program is to be experienced in conjunction with 'the what' of it, make for a welcome pedagogical inclusion [56].

To date, it is plausible that curricular time can be effectually used to introduce the skills and competencies needed for children to gain motor competence and fitness. However, creative means to facilitate other ways to participate are found to have been of value for children to use these meaningfully at their own discretion.

The 'I Can Resist' program takes explicit steps to build in structured choice and to facilitate peer support and self-agentic opportunities. Access in this regard shifts intended outcomes toward the facilitation of independent movers who can use, adapt and/or extend the resistance exercises into meaningful individual or group endeavours at their respective discretion ahead of motor proficiency outcomes. The latter progresses at the pace of each participant.

## 4. The 'I Can Resist' program

I Can Resist commences with resistance moves that are practised, refined and acquired through isometric challenges and then progressed through concentric-eccentric contractions and increase in number and complexity. The use of the 1st pronoun is to model and communicate and ensure the doing, and learning is done by each participant. That tactic also keeps the pace participant led. The spiral of progression (**Table 8**) reads from bottom to top and incorporates movement concepts so that participants have the opportunity to try the skills in a variety of ways that build understanding through interpretation of movement concepts. Mastery-wise, participants work their way through the bodyweight (only) progression spiral before they continue with added band resistance challenges. Further along the proficiency journey, participants can actually return (revisit) the progression spiral (**Table 8**. exemplification) and work their way through it incorporating resistance band challenges in ways found accessible and enjoyable. However, it is essential that participants work their way through the spiral managing only their own body weight first and foremost, before progressing onto the resistance movement skill series (**Tables 1** and **2**). Pedagogical tips are provided and discretional. They serve simply as a user-friendly optional guide. Clearly, this can be used and adapted to fit desired goals and expectations across a varied series of settings. The program has emerged from its original piloted three-step method incorporating the body, the resistance band and the suspension trainer as modes of improving biomotor fitness [57–59].

### 4.1 Health and safety guidelines

Health and safety remain consistent across each and all. Ensure respective health and safety policies and guidelines are adhered to across the planning and implementation and evaluation of program use. Participation remains student dependent and centred. Adapt to the known and emerging needs of the individual/group. Provide equitable, transparent and engaging ways the student can assist in your being effective in the provision and presentation of accessible learning opportunities. Rest and water breaks are also student centred and directed.

| | |
|---|---|
| • Body resistance progressions-body weight isometrics, dynamic body weight (Novice entry series without added band resistance *)<br>• I can lead a peer through a resistance movement set using any of the skills introduced and making sure lower, core and upper body being engaged.<br>• I can participate in peer-led resistance, move challenges, sequences and or games.<br>• I can participate in a mini challenge or game in my group, which includes 2–3 resistance moves (tutor guided and children can share ideas).<br>• I can show a partner my combo exercise routine and have them try it. I can try their routine.<br>• I can combo 2–3 exercises of my own choice to create a dynamic movement routine (e.g. lunge to line forwards, side lunges, back)<br>• I can travel from one point to another (about 5 meters) on all fours facing down, and then facing upwards<br>• I can perform a series of 5–8 superheroes (face down plane positions) using a coordinated and controlled proficient form<br>• I can perform a series of 3–5 V sits using legs bent or straight<br>• I can squat 5–10 times a stay balanced as I lower and stand up<br>• I can perform a series (5–10) of superheroes (plane positions) using proficient form and control<br>• I can perform a series of V sits (3–5) using proficient form and control<br>• I can perform a series (5–10) of curl-ups using proficient form and control<br>• I can hold a plank for a set target time (10–30 secs) and move my feet and then hands (one at a time) | Ready to transfer<br>In Progress<br>Attempting<br>Have students estimate how they are getting on progression spiral completion.<br>Any part can be revisited (and adapted), for example, completed on own, then with a partner, then with a group tying it with an added resistance band. Allow for motor creativity once motor skills have been acquired and how to use them understood.<br>No part of this is to be tested. This is a formative informal evaluation opportunity for students and tutors in knowing better where and when to adapt as and when needed. |

| |
|---|
| • I can hold a plane shape (facing downwards; superhero) keeping feet and arms off the ground<br>• I can start in a dish and move into a V shape, and hold a V shape (facing upwards) (3–5 secs)<br>• I can hold a dish shape (lying on floor, facing upwards) with feet and shoulders off the floor<br>• I can hold a sky-plank (facing upwards, keeping hips up) (5–10 secs)<br>• I can hold a side plank (both sides keeping my core tight) (5–10secs)<br>• I can hold a plank (facing downwards), in a straight form (and avoid a banana or bridge shape) (5–10 secs)<br>• I can curl up and hold (5–10 secs and /or show a peer) and return to the flat slowly<br>• I can hold a squat position and stay balanced (lower as if I am sitting on a chair, and stay there)<br>• I can push press my hands toward the ceiling (as if I am lifting and lowering a heavy boulder)<br>• I can lunge sideways (to right and to left)<br>• I can lunge backwards (right and left)<br>• I can get into a (static like a statue) a lunge position and hold it (10–20 secs)<br>• Novice resistance mover entry point using preferred mobility mode. (Participants more experienced in resistance exercise can aim to show greater control across the introductory lead into the program) |

**Table 8.**
*The 'I Can Resist' introductory progression spiral.*

### *4.1.1 Pedagogical tip*

*Fitness tip—do not make it about fitness! Keep it task/challenge oriented and match the language to show the genuine tutor focus of motor competence—agility development through balance and control.*

Inclusion target: Start somewhere, anywhere, for example, with a short 5–10 secs hold, and/or show a peer that takes even less but gets participants moving and trying and exploring and managing their bodies through a progression that takes them from high to medium and low levels, exploring personal space through basic moves, in a variety of ways. Progress using limited repetitions (or short-time bouts). That way peer modelling happens inadvertently and explicitly and attempts to stay task focused (rather than fitness). The way it is done.

*Can be revisited with a resistance band for the more experienced mover.

### *4.1.2 Pedagogical tip*

*Work your way through these by modelling and providing a brief explanation as you go. Keep all group members active and work your way up. Once you get to the top, start back again and repeat this time, change.*

**Table 8** depicts how the program is introduced. Explicit opportunities to develop motor competence manipulating the body in a variety of ways, at different levels to engage all major muscle groups are presented. Differing ways to develop social competence are integrated into the movement's challenges. Participants need to draw from cognitive, emotional and social skills to work their way through the progression spiral. The tutor initiates each new competence and skill through direct teaching and then facilitates greater inquiry-led challenges when students have something to access and try and something to talk about in their exchange.

Once participants have journeyed through the spiral, the resistance movement bank (**Tables 1** and **2**) can be utilised and drawn from to support the next progression spiral iterations. Tutors will want to show and tell each, as regards their utility, how they are done and exploring these across a variety of opportunities. If initiated from the outset of elementary years, a curriculum map can plot how and where and when the resistance skills, sequences and activities are interleaved into the full curriculum spiral, whereby competence, confidence and concomitant motor creativity are developmentally facilitated across a full six-year journey, for example. Tutors are well apt to make use of affordances as depicted through respective curricular and extracurricular chances.

### 4.2 Developmentally appropriate question—With or without bands?

Use the 'flag lunge' stability challenge across the sessions. If pupils struggle with this essential stability move (See formative assessment within item #3), provide band-free versions and as well as adapt as required. You can use any of the movement challenges from the resistance movement resource bank (#1–22). A worked example of how to use it following the movement induction is depicted in **Table 9**. Of course, this is but a linear rendition. Contextual educational topic choices with desired themes will readily modify if not replace this.

#### *4.2.1 Pedagogical replace*

*Have biomotor fitness as a by-product instead of the actual focus. Encore une fois—Do not make it about fitness! A progression learning spiral is exemplified and participants have patiently progressed through this. You have also shown patience with term use and modelled and explained how to get here. Take advantage of this.*

### 4.3 The 'I Can Resist' summary

Make it work for you and for your group. To be learned, it does need to be tried, understood and appreciated with plenty of chances to try and take calculated risks in figuring movement and verbal responses to challenges through less to more invariant opportunities.

### 4.4 Plenary

The premise behind 'I Can Resist' is that we, educators, can make resistance exercise meaningful and enjoyable for a wide variety of children and youth. One story that motivated the creation of this invitational approach remains with me today. One PE day, during a dedicated activity period of the lesson, a grade 4 student ran to me and was crying because he had never before felt his heart beating so hard through his

| Session | The B (main part of the session)<br>Use upper (U), core (C) and lower (L) exercises every session<br>Adapting options #7, #16 and #22 can be used every session-use/add as needed for your group | Check off | Notes |
|---|---|---|---|
| 3 | Lunge stability assessment<br>#1,#2, #3 (L) #10 (C), #19, #20 (U) | | Formative entry point<br>Student invitation to self-audit competence and understanding through the stability lunge challenge, then share with a peer. |
| 4 | #3, #5, #6 (L), #10, #12 (C), #13,#17,#18 (U) | | |
| 5 | #3, #4, (L) #? (L,C,U), #8 (C), #14, #15 (U) | | |
| 6 | #1, #2, #3 (L), #9, #12 (C), #19, #20,#15, #13 | | |
| 7 | #4, #5, #6 (L)#? (L, C, U), | | |
| 8 | #1, #3, #4 (L), #8, #9 (C), #11, #12, #13 (U) | | |
| 9 | #3 and group choice (L), #10 (C), #17, #18, #19, #20 (U) | | |
| 10 | #4, #2 (L), #? (L, C, U), Group choice (C), #15, #17 (U) | | |
| 11 | #1, #5, #6 (L), #14 (C,U), #21(L, C, U) | | |
| 12 | #3, #4 (L), #? (L, C, U), #19, #20, #15 (U) | | |
| 13 | #1, #2 (L), #8 or #9 (C), #11,#12,#13 (U) | | |
| 14 | #? (L, C, U), #21 (Choice combos) | | |
| 15 | #1, #2, #3 (L), #14, #15 (C), #12, #13, 17, #18 (U) | | |
| 16 | #4,#5,#6 (L), #8, #10 (C), #11, #13, #17 (U) | | |
| 17 | #1, #2, #3 (L), #21 (Core Choice combos), #19, #20 (U) | | |
| 18 | #1,#2.#3 (L), #? (L, C, U), #13, #17, #18 (U) | | |
| 19 | #1, #21 (Choice combos) | | |
| 20 | #1, #21(L combo), #21 (C combo) #21 (U combo), Group choice | | |
| 21 | #21(L combo), #21 (C combo) #21 (U combo), Group choice | | |
| 22 | Lunge stability assessment*<br>Group made L-C-U #21(with options) circuit<br>Into group designed small game, planned alongside emergent movement solutions and opportunities will be suitable.<br>You could use this formative field | | Formative exit point<br>How am I doing? What might I revisit?<br>How might I progress? |

| | |
|---|---|
| | assessment to top and tail your own scope and sequence, for example, a six-lesson medium-term plan—modify to fit as a means to inform students of their own progress and for you to be able to have this. |

*This exemplified scope and sequence follow the introductory body and self-management progression spiral (Table 3-content). It uses resistance movement vocabulary from **Tables 1** and 2. Students and educators can take ownership to use the movement vocabulary in a meaningful way to suit the intention and aspirations of the class and learning experience. Greater ownership and creativity can emerge using ideas such as those through the progression spiral challenge ideas (Table 3-pedagogical progression).*

**Table 9.**
*A basic rendition of starting resistance moves around the contextually relevant educational themes, topics and aims can be built.*

chest. I locked eyes with him, smiled and gently encouraged him to walk with me as his heart rate came down. I learned never again, to assume that all children are wired to move and move with vigour. The role of the other, the parent, the guardian and the peer, compelled me to develop means for children to become agentic alongside respective environmental factors, and hopefully irrespective of these where, and when they lacked opportunity for positive progression. The other part of my lesson learned of course is to make more efforts to offer joyful ways for the heart to soar and, educationally, to make this count. Now with my colleagues, we are able to progress such inclusive and aspirational practices in more accessible ways.

## Acknowledgements

Thank you, colleagues, for your commitment to building an array of valuable life skills and competencies through the bold implementation of the 'I Can Resist' in your own contexts, starting right from the beginning... My sincere thanks to colleagues and students from and found around the world, to my pole vault peer and my daughter for giving of their time to try out the program and capture these efforts in a simple and accessible way, as depicted in the start-up resistance movement bank (**Tables 1** and **2**). To my esteemed colleagues Dr. Kristy Howells and Dr. Pamela Murray for the next exciting and emerging steps as we take 'I Can Resist' and explore movement possibilities with our students as we build body strength, identity and belonging.

## Author details

Alison Morag Murray[1*], Pamela Murray[2] and Kristy Howells[3]

1 University of Roehampton, London, England

2 University of Worcester, London, England

3 Canterbury Christ Church University, London, England

*Address all correspondence to: alison.murray@roehampton.ac.uk

## References

[1] Graham G, Holt/Hale SA, Parker M, Hall T, Patton K. Children Moving, A Reflective Approach to Teaching Physical Education. 10th ed. New York: McGraw Hill; 2020

[2] Crocker PRE, Bouchard M, Gessaroli ME. Measuring enjoyment in youth sport setting: A confirmatory factor analysis of the Physical Activity Enjoyment Scale. Journal of Sport and Exercise Psychology. 1995;**17**:200-205

[3] Ryan RM, Deci EL. Self-determination theory and the facilitation of intrinsic motivation, social development, and well-being. American Psychologist. 2000;**55**(1):68-78. DOI: 10.1037/0003-066X.55.1.68

[4] Fletcher T, Ní C, Gleddie D, Beni SD. Meaningful Physical Education, an Approach for Teaching and Learning. Routledge Focus; 2022

[5] Viciana J, Mayorga-Vega D, Parra-Saldías M. Adolescents physical activity levels on physical education and non-physical education days according to gender, age, and weight status. *European Physical Education Review*. 2019;**25**(1):143-155. DOI: 10.1177/1356336X17706683

[6] Brudzynski L, Ebben W. Body image as a motivator and barrier to exercise participation. International Journal of Exercise Science. 2010;**3**(1):14-24. DOI: digitalcommons.wku.edu/ijes/vol3/iss1/3

[7] Thompson JK, Heinberg LJ, Altabe M, Tantleff-Dunn S. Exacting Beauty: Theory, Assessment, and Treatment of Body Image Disturbance. Washington, DC: American Psychological Association; 1999

[8] Vannucci A, McCauley Ohannessian C. Body image dissatisfaction and anxiety trajectories during adolescence. Journal of Clinical Child & Adolescent Psychology. 2018;**47**(5):785-795. DOI: 10.1080/15374416.2017.1390755

[9] Dion J, Blackburn M-E, Auclair J, Laberge L, Veillette S, Gaudreault M, et al. Development and aetiology of body dissatisfaction in adolescent boys and girls. International Journal of Adolescence and Youth. 2015;**20**(2):151-166

[10] Janssen I, Katzmarzyk PT, Srinivasan SR, Chen W, Malina RM, Bouchard C, et al. Combined influence of body mass index and waist circumference on coronary artery disease risk factors among children and adolescents. Pediatrics. 2005;**115**(6): 1623-1630. DOI: 10.1542/peds.2004-2588

[11] Coleman JC. The Nature of Adolescence. Routledge; 2011

[12] Schlüter C, Kraag G, Schmidt J. Body shaming: An exploratory study on its definition and classification. International Journal of Bullying Prevention. 2021. DOI: 10.1007/s42380-021-00109-3

[13] DeMet T, Wahl-Alexander Z. Integrating skill-related components of fitness into physical education. Strategies. 2019;**32**(5):10-17. DOI: 10.1080/08924562.2019.1637315

[14] Murray AM, Napper-Owen G. Metacognition, the METAPE-3, a new instructional model for physical education. In: Peters MA, editor. Encyclopedia of Teacher Education. Singapore: Springer; 2021. DOI: 10.1007/978-981-13-1179-6_421-1

[15] Phillips SM, Winett RA. Uncomplicated resistance training and health-related outcomes: Evidence for a

public health mandate. Current Sports Medicine Reports. 2010;**9**(4):208-213. DOI: 10.1249/JSR.0b013e3181e7da73

[16] Centers for Disease Control and Prevention. School health guidelines to promote healthy eating and physical activity. Morbidity and Mortality Weekly Report. 2011;**60**(5):1-76

[17] UNESCO. UNESCO International Charter of Physical Education and Sport, 21 November 1978. SHS/2015/PI/H/14 REV. 1978

[18] Department of Health & Social Care. UK Chief Medical Officers' Physical Activity Guidelines-GOV.UK. 2019. Available from: https://www.gov.uk/government/publications/physical-activity-guidelines-uk-chief-medical-officers-report

[19] Department of Health and Social Care. UK Chief Medical Officer's Physical Activity Guidelines. Department of Health and Social Care; 2019

[20] Jung H, Choi E. The importance of indirect teaching behaviour and its educational effects in physical education. Physical Education and Sport Pedagogy. 2014;**21**(2):1-16. DOI: 10.1080/17408989.2014.923990

[21] Office for Health Improvements and Disparities. Official Statistics. Obesity Profile: Statistical commentary. 2022. Available from: GOV.UK.https://www.gov.uk/government/statistics/obesity-profile-december-2022-update/obesity-profile-statistical-commentary-december-2022#

[22] Guthold R, Stevens GA, Riley LM, Bull FC. Global trends in insufficient physical activity among adolescents: A pooled analysis of 298 population-based surveys with 16 million participants. The Lancet Child & Adolescent Health. 2020;**4**(1):23-35. DOI: 10.1016/S2352-4642(19)30323-2

[23] Gabbard CP. Lifelong Motor Development. 8th ed. Wolters Kluwer Health; 2021

[24] O' Brien W, Belton S, Issartel J. The relationship between adolescents physical activity, fundamental movement skills and weight status. Journal of Sports Science. 2016;**34**(12): 1159-1167. DOI: 10.1080/02640414.2015.1096017

[25] Department for Education. National Curriculum in England: PE Programmes of Study. Department for Education; 2013

[26] SHAPE America. National Standards For Initial Health Education Teacher Education. Reston, VA: Author; 2018

[27] Association for Physical Education. Strategic Plan. 2015. Available from: https://www.afpe.org.uk/physical-education/strategic-plan

[28] Adeyemi-Walker LJ, Duncan M, Tallis J, Eyre E. Fundamental motor skills of children in deprived areas of England: A focus on age, gender and ethnicity. Children (Basel). 2018;**5**(8): 110. DOI: 10.3390/children5080110

[29] Stodden DF, Goodway JD, Langendorfer SJ, Roberton MA, Rudisill ME, Garcia C, et al. A developmental perspective on the role of motor skill competence in physical activity: An emergent relationship. Quest. 2008;**60**(2):290-306. DOI: 10.1080/00336297.2008.10483582

[30] Ovens A, Hopper T, Butler J. Complexity thinking in physical education. In: Ovens A, Hopper T, Buter J, editors. Reframing Curriculum, Pedagogy and Research. London: Routledge. Taylor & Francis Group; 2012

[31] Townsend N, Wickramasinghe K, Williams K, Bhatnagar P, Rayner M. Physical Activity Statistics 2015. London: British Heart Foundation; 2015

[32] HSS. U.S. Department of Health and Human Services: Office of Disease Prevention and Health Promotion—Healthy People 2010. Nasnewsletter. 2000;**15**(3):3

[33] Hobbs M, Daly-Smith A, McKenna J, Quarmby T, Morley D. Reconsidering current objectives for physical activity within physical education. British Journal of Sports Medicine. 2018;**52**(19):1229-1230. DOI: 10.1136/bjsports-2016-097328

[34] U.S. Department of Health and Human Services, editor. Physical Activity Guidelines for Americans. 2nd ed. U.S. Department of Health and Human Services; 2018

[35] Watkinson J, Causgrove Dunn J, Cavaliere N, Calzonetti K, Wilhelm L, Dwyer S. Engagement in playground activities as a criterion for diagnosing developmental coordination disorder. Adapted Physical Activity Quarterly, Human Kinetics Publishers Inc. 2001;**18**(1):18-34

[36] Hands B, Larkin D. Physical fitness differences in children with and without motor learning difficulties. European Journal of Special Needs Education. 2006;**21**(4):447-456

[37] Brunton G, Harden A, Rees R, Kavanagh J, Oliver S, Oakley A. Children and Physical Activity: A Systematic Review of Barriers and Facilitators. London: EPPI-Centre, Social Science Research Unit, Institute of Education, University of London; 2003 Available from: https://www.ncbi.nlm.nih.gov/books/NBK69896/

[38] Coleman KJ, Geller KS, Rosenkranz RR, Dzewaltowski DA. Physical activity and healthy eating in the after-school environment. Journal of School Health. 2008;**78**(12):633-640. DOI: 10.1111/j.1746-1561.2008.00359.x

[39] Diamond A, Lee K. Interventions shown to aid executive function development in children 4 to 12 years old. Science. 2011;**333**(6045):959-964. DOI: 10.1126/science

[40] Ofsted. Ofsted: Children Hardest Hit by COVID-19 (Coronavirus) Pandemic across the Sectors it Inspects and Regulates. Press release; 2020

[41] Adams S, Murray A. Primary physical education and its complex puzzle of diversity. In: Doull K, editor. Teaching a Diverse Primary Curriculum. London: Sage; 2022

[42] Prochaska JO, Norcross JC, DiClemente CC. Changing for Good: A Revolutionary Six-stage Program for Overcoming Bad Habits and Moving Your Life Positively Forward. New York, NY: Avon Books; 1994

[43] Gibson EJ. Perceiving the Affordances: A Portrait of Two Psychologists. 1st ed. Psychology Press; 2001. DOI: 10.4324/9781410604248

[44] O'Malley G, Thivel D. Physical activity and play in children who are obese. In: Frelut ML, editor. The ECOG's eBook on Child and Adolescent Obesity. 2015

[45] Robinson LE, Stodden DF, Barnett LM, Lopes VP, Logan SW, Rodrigues LP, et al. Motor competence and its effect on positive developmental trajectories of health. Sports Medicine. 2015;**45**:1273-1284. DOI: 10.1007/s40279-015-0351-6

[46] Luz C, Rodrigues LP, Meester A, Cordovil R. The relationship between

motor competence and health-related fitness in children and adolescents. PLoS One. 2017;**12**(6):e0179993. DOI: 10.1371/journal.pone.0179993

[47] Vygotsky LS. Mind in Society: The Development of Higher Psychological Processes. Cambridge, Mass.: Harvard University Press; 1978

[48] Powell K, Kalina C. Cognitive and social constructivism: Developing tools for an effective classroom. Education. 2009;**130**(2):241-250

[49] Bucher R. Diversity Consciousness: Opening our Minds to People, Cultures and Opportunities. 4th ed. Pearson Education; 2014. Available from: https://www.pearson.com/en-us/subject-catalog/p/diversity-consciousness-opening-our-minds-to-people-cultures-and-opportunities/P200000006981/9780137538669

[50] Ward N, Paul E, Watson P, Cooke GE, Hillman CH, Cohen NJ, et al. Enhanced learning through multimodal training: Evidence from a comprehensive cognitive, physical fitness, and neuroscience intervention. Scientific Reports. 2017;**7**(1):5808. DOI: 10.1038/s41598-017-06237-5

[51] Murray A, Kaitell E. Educational gymnastics. Embodiment of a constraint's agility approach. In: Griggs G, Randall V, editors. An Introduction to Primary Physical Education by. 2nd ed. Routledge; 2022

[52] Verschuren O, Ketelaar M, Gorter JW, Helders PJ, Uiterwaal CS, Takken T. Exercise training program in children and adolescents with cerebral palsy: A randomized controlled trial. Archives of Pediatrics & Adolescent Medicine. 2007;**161**(11):1075-1081. DOI: 10.1001/archpedi.161.11.1075

[53] Plowman SA, Meredith MD, editors. Fitnessgram/Activitygram Reference Guide. 4th ed. Dallas, TX: The Cooper Institute; 2013

[54] Sperling RA, DuBois N, Howard BC, Staley R. Metacognition and self-regulated learning constructs. Educational Research and Evaluation. 2004;**1**(2):117-139. DOI: 10.1076/edre.10.2.117.27905

[55] Office for Health Improvement & Disparities. Official Statistics. NCMP Changes in the Prevalence of Child Obesity Between 2019 to 2020 and 2020 to 2021. Office for Health Improvement & Disparities; 2022

[56] Murray A, Murray P, Woods G, Howells K, McKenna J. The complexities of developing motor competence through a health and skill related programme. Developing student agency through developmentally appropriate resistance. In: International Motor Development Research Consortium. Advancing Motor Development Research in the 21st Century Virtual Conference. South Carolina, USA; 2020

[57] Murray AM. Skill and fitness related development via metacognitive instruction. Physical Education Matters. 2013;**8**(2):59-64

[58] Murray AM, Murray-Hopkin PF. Developmentally appropriate health and skill related fitness training in physical education. Physical Education Matters. 2014;**9**(1):62-67

[59] Murray AM, Murray P, Woods G, Patel B, Palouseo J. Developmentally appropriate resistance training in physical education. American Alliance for Health, Physical Education and Dance. Strategies, a Journal for Physical and Sport Educators. 2013;**26**(2):23-29

Section 2

# Medicine

Chapter 3

# Resistance Training is Medicine: Stay Active and Reap the Reward, Live in your Life!

*Endang Ernandini and William Giovanni Mulyanaga*


## Abstract

The world of physical medicine and rehabilitation still believes that exercise is medicine. Muscle mass will naturally decrease with aging, 3–8% every decade after a person turns 30 years old, getting worse over the age of 50 years, which is 5–10% every decade. Some studies state that for healthy people, resistance training (RT) performed 2–3 times per week with 12–20 total sets of exercises will add muscle mass. The addition of 1.4 kg of muscle mass was accompanied by the disappearance of about 1.8 kg of fat. RT plus aerobic exercises (AE) complemented with caloric resistance (CR) can result in a reduction of 5.1 kg or 7.1% of fat. Some research papers state that for stable CAD patients starting with 3 months of AE followed by an RT program of 40–60% intensity 1x RM, 1–2 sets, 8–10 repetitions, 2–3 days per week, duration not more than 60 minutes. Recommendation for a person with intellectual disability can be simple and harmless RT tools. The prescription for COVID-19 survivors consists of AE for 5 to 30 minutes with low to moderate intensity, plus 1–2 sets of RT, 8–10 reps at 30–80% 1xRM.


**Keywords:** resistance training, exercise, medicine, special condition, prescription

## 1. Introduction

Resistance training (RT) is part of several types of exercises that can be recommended as one of the lifestyles and has a positive effect on a person's health status [1]. This is one of the exercises that should be done together with other exercises that will form or maintain endurance, balance, flexibility, and strength. Blending these four types of exercises is very important to maintain optimal health and to be able to carry out optimal activities in daily life. Strength training is a form of exercise that focuses on the use of weights or resistance to build muscles, as well as ligaments and bones, increase power, and maintain posture [2].

RT, also known as weight training or strength training, is a physical activity to improve neuromuscular and musculoskeletal fitness and physical performance by training muscles or a group of muscles, which is done by resisting weights from the outside [1, 3, 4]. External load can be in form of disc, barbells, dumbbells, and resistance bands. Folland et al., 2007 [5] and Spiering et al., 2008 [6] state that physical exercise using some kind of resistance exercise can also be incorporated into the

RT [5, 6]. Resistance training can also be performed by using body weight, such as push-ups and squats [1].

The first question that arises is "What is the main purpose of doing this RT activity as the chosen type of sport instead of doing other types of exercises?" It has been proven by many studies and articles that RT can produce a state of muscle hypertrophy [3–6] and produce additional muscle endurance, muscle strength, maximum strength, muscle explosion, and power [4, 7, 8]. In addition to the ability of RT to create muscle hypertrophy, it is also able to create functional additions to the body, besides only the esthetic function of body shape, which we will learn more about in the next chapter.

In contrast to aerobic exercise, which already has standards that are widely accepted in society, RT still needs to be studied for its needs and advantages for the various physical circumstances of a person who will do it, especially people with special conditions. The best procedure for identifying the most adequate and optimal RT exercises is through careful experimentation as well as observations and experiences. Through experiments, observations, and experiences, it can be analyzed and concluded how to obtain a method, a formulation for the dose of load applied to improve the state of health and even improve the quality of life of a person. RT is also expected to be applied not only to healthy individuals but also to individuals with certain health conditions. Suchomel et al., 2018 [9] also DeWeese et al., 2015 [10] remind us that: 1) it is necessary to pay attention to the selection of exercises to produce a balance between determining and using the weight of the load as well as its preparations to achieve the specified goals, 2) management of fatigue begins from anticipating the possibility of overtraining to carrying out rest procedures, and 3) it is necessary to pay attention to the right stages and timing to produce good performance [3, 9, 10].

## 2. Physiology of exercise

Exercise forces the body to do more movement compared to when resting. Movement during exercise stimulates the sympathetic nervous system and will increase the body's response integrally. This response is necessary for the body to maintain hemostasis over the increased metabolism of the heart, lungs, muscles, brain, and other organs [11].

### 2.1 Cardiovascular system response

Physiologists say that when a person performs a heavy physical activity, the muscles only show 30% of their maximal capacity, while the respiratory and cardiovascular systems have reached much higher activity, 60% and 90% of their maximal capacity, respectively. Based on this data and information, some physiologists state that the greatest factor affecting the transportation of O2 and nutrients to the muscles that will support metabolism in aerobic exercise is the cardiovascular system. Thus, the exercise is aimed mainly to improve cardiovascular efficiency [2, 12, 13]. The increase in endurance levels of the cardiorespiratory system is not solely produced by AE but also RT. RT helps to add endurance values in cycling (47%), walking (38%), and running (12%) activities. The increase in this value is not due to an increase in the value of VO2max, but mainly because of the increase in fatigue threshold. This can occur due to the recruitment of muscle cells and mitochondria, so we can say that cardiorespiratory endurance is also affected by muscle strength in addition to muscle endurance [14].

### 2.2 Muscle response

The human body has three types of muscle tissue: skeletal muscle, smooth muscle, and special muscle, called the cardiac muscle. As the name implies, most skeletal muscles are attached to skeletal bones, and they have the main function for active movement [2]. Skeletal muscles make up most of the body mass, it is estimated to be about 40% of body mass in total. Tendon is further classified into two parts, one part is immobile and attached closer to the torso, called origo. The other part of a tendon can relatively move and is attached farther to the body, called insersio [2].

What requirements are needed to move the skeleton? How can muscles move the skeleton? The answer is by contracting. The muscle contraction will bring the bone closer or away according to the condition. The movement is possible due to the presence of joints, which connect the bones. The driving muscle is called the flexor when the task is to bring the two bones connected to the joint closer, and the movement is called flexion. In contrast, when the contraction of the skeletal muscle drives the two bones away, the muscle is called extensor and the movement is called extension. The flexor muscle will be paired with the extensor muscle, and together they are called antagonist muscle group. The task of these antagonist muscles is to move closer and further from the fulcrum point. Contracting alternately, relaxing alternately. The coordinated movement between these muscles allows us to do daily activities effectively [15].

Active muscle contraction requires a supply of energy coming from adenosine triphosphate (ATP), while relaxation of the muscle is a state of relinquishment from a state of contraction. Muscle movement always requires energy, both when contracting and relaxing. When contracting, muscles need energy to move interlocking. When relaxing, muscle requires energy to pump $Ca2+$ ions back into the sarcoplasmic reticulum, and also to return $Na$ + ions to extracellular and $K+$ ions to intracellular [15].

Where do muscles get energy (ATP) from to perform their duties? Can muscles run out of ATP? The amount of ATP energy available in the muscle fibers is only enough to do about 8 to 10 wrinkles. As the source of energy stored in the muscle, it is very limited in quantity. Muscles must use other sources of energy to still be able to carry out their duties, that is to transfer energy from chemical bonds stored in nutrients into ATP. Carbohydrates, especially glucose, are the fastest and most efficient sources of energy. Glucose molecules will produce 30 ATP when metabolized using oxygen (called aerobic metabolism). However, when the oxygen supply is exhausted, this metabolism will enter the anaerobic process, which only produces 2 ATP. Muscles also get energy from fatty acids, which also always require oxygen, and this process is relatively slow. Skeletal muscles in carrying out their tasks still prefer to rely on glucose. Protein is also not a major producer of energy sources for muscle contraction, preferably used for cell repair [15].

### 2.3 Hormones response

The fundamental difference in physiology exercises can be seen from gender differences, where the hormone testosterone gives the different characteristics in males and females. This hormone has a more influential role for males in exercise in terms of increasing male muscle mass. Besides testosterone, it turns out that there are many other hormones that are affected and affecting the ability to carry out the exercise as well as in terms of the results of the exercise. Gharahdaghi et al., 2021 [16] mentioned that the body during exercise requires work initiated by these hormones, especially when we talk about maintaining and even developing muscle mass as a goal of exercising. Hormones such as testosterone, estrogen, growth hormone (GH), and insulin-like growth factor (IGF) have a role in the success of an exercise [16].

Hooper et al., 2017 [17] stated that muscle contraction exercises in RT remain the leading major role in muscle hypertrophy through the formation of muscle protein synthesis (MPS) [17]. This response is controlled by the combination of weight training and the associated hormone release. Skeletal muscle mass, which at least comprises 40–45% of the entire body mass, will be preserved from sarcopenia problems caused by aging [18].

The RT pathway of inducing an anabolic response to the skeletal muscles can be traced from several studies and statements from experts in the field. RT will stimulate the work of thc hormone testosterone, GH, and estrogen (in accordance with the rhythm of the body of a menstrual woman), as well as IGF. Basically, stimulation of these hormones functions to repair the damaged cells that occur in the muscles while doing exercises. Owing to the balanced work between MPS and muscle protein breakdown (MPB), muscle cells can be repaired, maintained, and developed to increase muscle fiber [16].

The release of testosterone is induced by exercise, both acutely and chronically (as exercise becomes a habit of life), and affected by sex and age. Hooper et al. stated that in the acute phase of exercising, the level of serum testosterone rises from 13 (resting level) to 38 (in 30 minutes) $nmol.L^{-1}$. Then it will decrease back to the baseline immediately after finishing the exercise [17]. If this exercise becomes a habit of life, it is not impossible that this phenomenon will play a very long role in the development and growth of muscles. This is reinforced by statements from Hansen et al., 2001 [18] and Ahtiainen et al., 2003 [19], where they confirmed that after 9 weeks of RE, the level of serum of these hormones was found to be increased steadily, leading to even more optimal muscle growth [18, 19]. There are authors who also state that the role of testosterone response and adaptation of exercise in women must still be tested and studied further.

Hermansen et al., 2017 [20] stated that the physiological increment of GH values after doing RT is basically adding protein synthesis, which also has the ability to repair muscle tissue and also affects muscle mass without affecting the ability to function muscles [20]. It was also reported that there was a correlation between RT stimulating an increase in GH and the presence of muscle hypertrophy of type I and II muscle fiber types [21].

RT also provides a rapid response to an increase in systemic levels of IGF-1 from 45 (resting state) to 65 nM when performing RT and returning to the baseline after completing RT. Ogasawara et al., 2016 [22] stated that this situation is also alleged to be an important thing in muscle growth [22]. Likewise, the statement of Bjersing et al., 2017 [23], who proved the existence of an increase in muscle strength after doing RT by taking into account IGF-1 levels [23]. Similar to the influence of GH, the role of IGF-1 will stimulate a pathway that will improve the state of muscle hypertrophy, which also greatly affects the absorption of glucose into the muscles to be able to produce available energy for the continuation of the active movement of muscles [24].

### 2.4 Fats metabolism response

Research explains that after 30 minutes from the start of physical exercise, particularly aerobic, the concentration of free fatty acids in the blood will increase significantly. That is, at that 30th minute, the fat will be mobilized from the adipose tissue. However, the process of breaking down these fatty acids is slower than glucose metabolism through the glycolysis process, so the energy production that occurs in the muscles is both from fatty acids and glucose. In lower-intensity and aerobic physical exercise, the largest source of energy production, ATP, comes from fat with a time of more than 30 minutes, while during medium–high-intensity physical exercise, the main source of energy is carbohydrates [2].

## 3. Resistance training is medicine

RT is now publicly known, not necessarily only applicable to athletes, such as weightlifters, bodybuilders, and footballers. In these sports, athletes are demanded to have much higher muscle strength or be esthetically pleasing for competitions. However, people in general do not have a reason to do RT, especially people with certain medical conditions. Fear and disbelief, despite of popularity of RT, still do not make RT a part of everyday life [25]. The world of physical medicine and rehabilitation still believes that exercise is medicine. Many authors implement endurance exercise as a therapeutic exercise for patients with stroke, heart disease, and DM while emphasizing RT for patients with postinjury. Nowadays, some of the authors, through their experience and personal daily clinical observations, began to show the courage to choose RT as a type of therapeutic exercise for patients with certain diseases. Prescription of RT as a medicine seems to have more advantages than disadvantages, when done carefully and full of caution (always looking at the patient's response and vital signs).

Muscle mass will naturally decrease with aging, 3–8% every decade after a person turns 30 years old. Flack et al. and Frontera et al. stated that at least 0.2 kg of muscle is lost annually [26, 27]. Marcell also gives even more surprising data for muscle mass loss over the age of 50 years, which is 5–10% every decade [28]. Nelson et al. [29] stated that muscle mass was close to 0.4 kg per year [29]. Skeletal muscles that weigh about 40% of our body have a role in burning glucose and triglyceride, so losing muscle mass will increase glucose intolerance. Even in untrained muscles, skeletal muscles are responsible for a massive overhaul and synthesis of proteins. This overhauling metabolism will be responsible for calorie expenditure needed even at rest. Calories that must be prepared for this metabolic process have values ranging from 11 to 12 $cal.d^{-1}.kg^{-1}$ [30]. One can imagine the disadvantages of losing muscle that occurs both due to sarcopenia and sedentary lifestyle. Inactive living habits will decrease muscle mass, which will lead to a decrement in the metabolic rate of the body. A decrease in metabolic rate will lead to the growth of body fat tissue, especially intraabdominal fat. The accumulation of fat and the reduction of muscle mass will certainly have an impact on decreasing metabolic rates. This condition will occur as a cyclic process and affect one another, becoming the so-called vicious circle. Efforts are needed to break the loop, and according to some studies it turns out that RT can give quite promising answers.

Some studies state that RT exercises performed 2–3 times per week with 12–20 total sets of exercises will add muscle mass in all adults in a wide age range. The addition of an average of 1.4 kg of muscle mass occurs after performing 3 months of RT. It can be concluded that RT helps restore muscle mass gain, even in nonathlete population. The addition of 1.4 kg of muscle mass was accompanied by the disappearance of about 1.8 kg of fat [31–34]. The research become more interesting because it showed a reduction in abdominal adipose fat tissue in elderly women who do RT, not just a reduction in abdominal fat in elderly men. Participants who regularly do RT for 2 years were able to remove 2/3 of intra-abdominal fat, compared to the participants who did not do exercise [35–38]. Hurley et al. [39] believe that the addition of metabolic rates, even at rest, plays a major role in increasing insulin sensitivity and sympathetic nerve activation, two of many factors affecting intraabdominal fat accumulation. The addition of metabolic rate is an intraabdominal fat loss factor with this calculation: if RT is done twice per week for 20 minutes each day, it will be close to the energy use of 5000 calories per month [39].

In a study of nursing home residents (with an average age of 89 years), the participants performed 1 set of exercises of RT with 6 machines twice per week for 14 weeks. At the end of this study, an evaluation was obtained and the results of the analysis found that all the participants increased their muscle strength by 60%, with the addition of 1.7 kg of muscle mass as well as a functional increase in independence by 14 [25].

## 4. Prescription of resistance training for healthy people, what do we want to achieve?

The Canadian Physical Activity Guidelines 2011 have recommended aerobic exercise and training as excellent things to do to add health value. This applies to all healthy people aged 18 to 64, even to people over the age of 65. This recommendation states that one person should do at least 150 minutes of exercise in a week (7 days). They recommend moderate to vigorous intensity exercise. They also add that it will be better if a person continues to do RT to maintain muscle and bone strength by exercising groups of major muscles at least twice a week [1].

A systematic review of selected 11 studies with 382,627 participants, from 2009 to 2019, looked for facts by comparing two large groups, the intervention group doing RT and the group that does not do RT. In the group that performed RT, it was recorded and statistically proven that there was a correlation between doing RT and reduction of death for any reason, decrease in the occurrence of cardiovascular disease, and increase in physical functional capacity. The effects related to cognitive function are not yet clear, they must be further proven. Unwanted side effects were not consistently monitored or reported in these studies. However, it is stated that there are no serious or injurious side effects or uncommon side effects. Overall, RT is beneficial in improving the health status of adults and the benefits outweigh the disadvantages [40].

RT can be a fun exercise with a variety of tools with certain weights. RT can also be done simply by relying on one's own body weight with certain movements that resist the force of gravity. In line with the advancement of RT technology, it can be done using machines and even robotic tools that can be programmed and adjusted to one's needs and abilities. If the advance tools are not available, we can make simple tools with simple materials around us. For instance, we can make a load from a used mineral water drinking bottle filled with fine sand. Determine the weight of the tool load we need.

No matter how healthy a person is, try to determine the RT load and the practice prescribing method with an initial test first. This initial data can be used as a reference for a basic or initial program and can be used to evaluate the progress of the program being trained. As one of the suggestions for training and achieving a defined goal, no matter how much your target load is, start by practicing multi-joint involving large muscles and then train by involving a single joint targeting more focused muscles.

Here is the RT reference taken from ACSM:

See **Table 1.**

To achieve the optimal goal of RT, there are 4 factors that should be considered, namely muscle strength, muscle power, muscle hypertrophy, and local muscle endurance. These four factors can be developed if the RT prescription is tailor-made, determined and carried out according to the needs and capabilities. RT prescription should always consider the load, volume, rest period between sets, and frequency of each exercise.

1. Load: how heavy it should be lifted based on how much % 1xRM.

2. Volume: total how many kinds of exercises (muscle groups trained), how many sets in each kind of movement, and how many reps in each set.

3. Rest time: the distance of resting time from one movement to another.

4. Frequency: the number of days on which training sessions are conducted each week.

See **Table 2.**

Frequency can be done by considering the reference as follows:

1. When you do it all together (upper as well as lower body) at once, you can do it two to three times per week, per muscle group.

2. If you do it separately, for example, upper body only, other days lower body only; you can do it up to four times per week.

3. An athlete can do it 4–6 times per week because they do have the ability and goals to win the competition.

| | **Free-Weight** | **Machine-Based** | **Body Weight** |
|---|---|---|---|
| Chest | Supine Bench Press | Seated Chest Press | Push-ups |
| Back | Bent-over Barbell Rows | Lat Pulldown | Pull-ups |
| Shoulder | Dumbbell Lateral Raise | Shoulder Press | Arm Circles |
| Biceps | Barbell/ Dumbbell Curls | Cable Curls | Reverse Grip Pull-ups |
| Triceps | Dumbbell Kickbacks | Pressdowns | Dips |
| Abdomen | Weighted Crunches | Seated “Abs” Machine | Crunches. Prone Planks |
| Quadriceps | Back Squats | Leg Extension | Body Weight Lunges |
| Hamstring | Stiff-leg Deadlifts | Leg Curls | Hip-ups |

**Table 1.**
*American College of Sports Medicine. Copyright © 2013 American College of Sports Medicine. This brochure was created by Michael R. Esco, Ph.D., HFS, CSCS*D, It is a product of ACSM's Consumer Information Committee. Visit ACSM online at www.acsm.org [41].*

| No. | Goal | Exercise level | Loading | Vol: exercise x set x repetition | Resting between |
|---|---|---|---|---|---|
| 1a. | Muscle strength | Intermediate | 60–70% | (6–8) x (1–3) x (8–12) | 2–3 min |
| 1b. | | Advance | 80–100% | (6–8) x (2–6) x (1–8) | 1–2 min |
| 2a. | Muscle power | Upper body | 30–60% | (3–4) x (1–3) x (3–6) | 2–3 min heavy load |
| | | | | | 1–2 min easy load |
| 2b. | | Lower body | 0–60% | (3–4) x (1–3) x (3–6) | 2–3 min heavy load |
| | | | | | 1–2 min easy load |
| 3a. | Hypertrophy muscle | Intermediate | 70–85% | (6–8) x (1–3) x (8–12) | 2–3 min heavy load |
| | | | | | 1–2 min easy load |
| 3b. | | Advance | 70–100% | (6–8) x (3–6) x (1–12) | 2–3 min heavy load |
| | | | | | 1–2 min easy load |
| 4. | Local Muscle Endurance | | Max 70% | @muscle group x (2–4) x (10–25) | 30 sec – 1 min |

**Table 2.**
*American College of Sports Medicine. Copyright © 2013 American College of Sports Medicine. This brochure was created by Michael R. Esco, Ph.D., HFS, CSCS*D. it is a product of ACSM's consumer information committee. Visit ACSM online at www.acsm.org [41]. Modified by Ernandini*

Beware of overtraining. Overtraining can occur because the interventions carried out are exceeding the capabilities of the individual. Symptoms of overtraining in RT can be severe pain, injuries to muscles, joints, tendons, or heavy fatigue. This can be triggered by exceedingly heavy load, too many muscles being exercised, too many repetitions, or doing RT too often. Injuries also often occur because we misposition our posture with the weight that must be lifted. It is best to do the exercise in tiered, gradual, and continuous manner instead of a sudden increment of loads [41]. Ernandini et al. [42] stated that the most important thing is safety in doing exercise, so do an MCU to find out your fitness level medically first [42].

## 5. Resistance training as ammunition to combat obesity

The status of obesity is believed to be increasing along with the improving economy, especially in countries with high per capita income. The incidence of obesity is also undeniably caused due to modern lifestyle. Obesity is also believed and proven to be a contributing to DM and cardiovascular and cancer diseases [43]. In this journal, it is also stated that the role of regulating the amount and type of food and exercise will help calorie deficit. A 5% weight loss can add significant value to the improvement of health status and cardiovascular health function [44, 45].

Some studies look for the answers to whether RT plays a role in preventing obesity status over a long period, as well as RT's usage as an exercise to reduce obesity cases. So far, AE has been accepted to help maintain weight and prevent obesity. A systematic review using the prospective cohort study in 2021 involved 11.938 participants [43]. In this study, obesity is defined as BMI results ≥30 kg/m$^2$ [46], waist circumference (wc) > 102 cm for men and > 88 cm for women [47], and percent body fat (PBF) ≥ 25% and 30% for men and women, respectively. This study included 11,938 adult participants who were not obese and were followed for 6 years. After taking into account several factors that may affect the results of this study such as age, sex, examination year, smoking, alcohol consumption, hypertension, hypercholesterolemia, and DM, the results show that RT will affect at least 20–30% of participants [48] in reducing the risk of becoming obese for the next 6 years [43]. Of course, with a strong commitment to maintaining a healthy lifestyle to maintain BB and ideal body composition to support health.

The main goal of a healthy lifestyle is to maintain good health status. By living a healthy lifestyle, one can get pleasant side effects in the form of balanced body weight and composition. However, in this super comfortable and easy era, it is a challenge for one to keep his body in optimal condition. Until now, it is still believed that the decrease in the amount of visceral fat and subcutaneous fat is very important and can decrease the incidence of metabolic cardiovascular diseases such as DM, heart attacks, and strokes. Obesity can now be considered a threat to the medical world because it is not only esthetically unpleasing but also a risk factor leading to comorbidities as explained above.

Several studies that chose RT as an exercise to combat obesity were collected and analyzed in a systematic review. Electronic data collection from various studies taken till December 2020, recorded 4184 people with obesity and overweight. This study involved participants aged <18 years, >18–35 years, >35–59 years, and ≥ 60 years, which were given exercise as an intervention for at least four weeks. The types of interventions they carried out further differed into RT alone (49.1%), RT + AE (44%), RT + restriction calorie (RC) (5.3%), and RT + AE + RC (7%). The average treatment was 14.6 weeks of exercise, with a frequency of 1 to 5x/week and variety of intensities of RT (low, moderate, and heavy). Outcome measures were the calculation of body fat, fat mass, visceral adipose tissue (VAT), and subcutaneous adipose (SAT), including body weight and BMI as secondary outcomes [49].

The results of RT alone actually already have a significant difference statistically, but the change value is categorized as small to moderate when analyzed statistically. RT alone has a significant enough role to increase muscle mass weight. RT alone can reduce 2.2% of fat or 1.6 kg of fat [49].

SR conducted by Xinhong Liu et al. 2022 involved 15 studies with a total of 669 subjects, observing three types of exercise in RT: own body weight (OBW), resistance bands (RB), and free weight (FW). It is concluded that RB is the most effective tool in RT for fat removal in cases of overweight and obese. RB has a much more flexible form and work than using certain loads. RB is more adjustable and can follow shape of the body. The pull of RB will provide tensile force that will increase along with the elongation of RB. The intensity of this RB tensile force will not be too high, so the body can do its work more slowly with a lower intensity and the body will use aerobic oxidation, which will use glucose and fat as main source of energy [50, 51]. RB is flexible and can follow the direction of the pulling force following a group of muscles used for the movement, and this will greatly help fat burning. However, because the intensity of RB is not high, the stimulation in the muscles will not continue, hence the muscle mass formation will not be optimal. In addition, the light RB will not have a heavy impact, especially on the joints of overweight and obese [50].

When reviewed further, there are more types of exercises and interventions, which also give meaningful results in combating obesity. Multicomplex exercises turned out to have better results since each intervention had its own role. It is necessary to give monitored, implementable, measurable, accountable, and safe prescriptions to achieve optimal results. These results will be even better when RT is complemented by a reduction in the calories. RT + CR exercises will reduce fat by 3.8%. An encouraging result is when RT plus AE exercises, complemented with CR, can result in a reduction of 5.1 kg of fat, or 7.1%. This effect remains consistent for adolescents to the elderly, with the greatest number of meaningful changes in young adulthood. Decrease in VAT and SAT obtained from multicomplex therapy consisting of RT + AE + RC. Meaningful change with a fairly satisfactory value remains consequential at all ages, even postmenopausal women [49].

*Garrow and Sumerbell* predict that a 20–30% rcduction in body weight caused by CR alone in adults is not due to a reduction in fat mass. For this reason, more than just CR efforts are needed for overweight and obesity reduction programs [52]. In line with the study, Sardeli et al. [53] stated RT is required to build skeletal muscle as much as 1.8 kg. When skeletal muscles contract, especially during exercises, our body will release myokine, myostatin, interleukin 6 (IL-6), and brain-derived neutrophic factor (BDNF). These substances will provide protection for the body against adipokines proinflammatory in obese bodies. The formation of muscles plays an important role in increasing resting energy expenditure, which leads to a decrement in obesity and overweight status [53].

## 6. Prescription resistance training for Cardiovascular Disease (CVD)

Hypertension (HBP) is one of nine risk factors leading to CVD. HBP is estimated to cause >7 million deaths annually, 13% of total deaths worldwide [54]. Meta-analysis by Lewington in 2002 stated that the safe blood pressure to be free from the threat of disease and death from CVD is at 115/75 mmHg [55]. On that basis, adequate blood pressure management must be socialized to the community to become a worldwide self-monitoring. Adequate BP control is closely related to life habits, including weight control, moderate intake of alcohol, a diet of fresh fruits and vegetables, reducing saturated fat, and staying active in daily life and exercise [55, 56]. So far, there have been many studies and writings that recommend aerobic exercise such as: walking, jogging, and cycling for controlling and even lowering BP on HBP. This is the time to consider one type of exercise that has an effect on metabolic health as well as in the preventive efforts of CVD [55, 57].

Several studies collected in a meta-analysis show several things about the effect of RT on BP on subject groups that have undergone RT and non-RT groups. This research was conducted from 1987 to June 2010. Based on the type of contraction, RT is also divided into two more groups: RT dynamic and RT static/isometric. Dynamic RT consists of concentric and eccentric contraction by moving an arm or leg that causes the length and tension of muscles and tendons to change. Meanwhile, static RT is a state of contraction against the load by not moving or not extending or stretching muscles or tendons. After 16 weeks of exercise, the subjects were then evaluated and compared to their initial values. To eliminate bias, the subjects were instructed not to change their lifestyles during this time while carrying out the pre-ordered exercise, which is a dynamic RT or static RT, according to their group. The result was then analyzed and it was found that from the two groups, dynamic RT exercises with moderate intensity, as well as low intensity in static RT, had a decreasing BP systole and BP diastole significantly. It was also noted that the dynamic RT group also had a good effect on things that are predictor CVD risk factors, such as increase in VO2pea and decrease in body fat and plasma triglyceride. The results of the analysis in this study can be concluded to have a clinical meaning that a decrease in SBP and DBP in a resting state even though it is only 3 mmHg can reduce the risk of CAD 5%, stroke 8% and other deaths by as much as 4% [54].

The increase in mortality in chronic CVD such as hypertension and diabetes is often associated with arterial stiffness. This stiffness results from the loss of elastic fibers and the accumulation of stiff collagen debris attached to the arterial wall. This stiffness results from the loss of elastic fibers and the accumulation of stiff collagen debris attached to the arterial wall. Many studies have found that this stiffness is strongly related to a person's physical activity. Activities such as walking and running, affect in a positive way to prevent vascular stiffness. The next question will be, whether RT affects arterial stiffness in positive or negative manner? A meta-analysis tried to answer this question, involving 981 participants aged 18 to 88, and they were divided into experimental groups and control groups. The intervention group carried out RT for 8 to 12 weeks with a frequency of 1 to 5 times per week, with intensity ranging from 30 to 90% 1RM. All subjects were measured for their carotid, femoral, tibial, and brachial arterial pulse rates. In conclusion, RT has no effect on the speed of arterial waves. The researchers did not stop there, they carried out a regression analysis to see the involvement of each parameter. After performing a regression analysis, it was found that only the intensity of exercise had a correlation with the change in the speed of the arterial wave rate. Light to moderate intensity significantly reduces the speed of arterial wave beating, while high intensity has no meaningful effect. Then the researchers also continued the regression analysis of age, then found that the barrier was seen meaningfully in subjects with an age of more than 40 years. Researchers then concluded that RT with mild to moderate intensity meaningfully decreases arterial stiffness in groups over 40 and also has a moderate correlation in those under 40 years of age [57].

The increase in the rate of arterial waves of 1 m/s alone will increase the risk factor of CVD by around 12–14% and the mortality rate by 13–15%. Although it is asserted that RT with mild and moderate intensity will have a good impact on the prevention and improvement of arterial stiffness, the exact explanation of it has not been obtained satisfactorily. Researchers made a hypothesis that states that RT with an intensity of 30–70% will activate only a small amount of the sympathetic nervous system, so it will not increase muscle tone. This has a beneficial effect on the blood circulation system by increasing endothelial function [57].

*Haslan et al.* [58] reported that CAD patients with mild hypertension were declared safe doing RT with an intensity of 40–60% 1xRM [58]. Recommendation for safe rehabilitation program for stable CAD patients without complaints starting with 3 months of AE followed by an RT program of 40–60% intensity 1x RM, 1–2 sets, 8–10 repetitions, 2–3 days per week, duration not more than 60 minutes. There is no recurrence of symptoms and it is shown to increase muscular strength and endurance [59]. Especially for postoperative patients with cardiac and post-myocardial infraction (MI) cases, it is recommended to postpone RT by at least 4 to 6 months [60, 61]. RT should be done progressively, starting low and gradually increasing until a certain goal.

If you are going to do isometric RT, do a mild one. Because isometric movement means making the same muscle contraction without moving the joint so that there is no extension of the length of the muscle involved, causing a disproportionate increase in blood pressure [14].

## 7. Recommendation and effects of RT for intellectual disability of people

There are not many studies about RT programs for adults with intellectual impairments (ID). They often have intellectual problems as well as emotional problems, although many of them also have adequate gross motor ability. According to American Psychiatric Association, ID is a disorder due to deficit in person's cognition as well as a disorder in the concept of thinking, which certainly has an impact on practical matters in social activity, and this condition is diagnosed before the age of 18 years [61]. Several studies done by Dairo et al. [62] and Harris L et al. [63] reported that IDs are a group of people who are at risk of injury and tend to have a sedentary lifestyle, which increases the risk for cardiovascular disease, hypertension, obesity, and DM [62, 63].

The lower the IQ, the lower the ability to record memory. Their ability to concentrate and communicate can also be seriously lacking, so monitoring by training instructors and caregivers is still very necessary. Safety remains a major issue for individuals with intellectual disability in doing exercise [64].

The guidelines for prescribing RT from ACSM must still be maintained to obtain excellent health quality. RT is still sought to involve at least 6 to 8 large muscle groups, performed by involving both multi joints and single joint. Possibilities have to be considered: how about exercise using muscle contraction (either eccentric and concentric), also isotonic, isometric and isokinetic exercise, and also exercise using equipment.

A systematic review observation consisting of several studies, involving 280 subjects who had an IQ below 70 with an average age of 18.23 years ±2.86 years, wanted to see how the prescribing and effects of RT for IDs. Interventions performed were varying duration of RT with an average of 12 weeks, 2–5 times a week. All the studies involved gave encouraging results by showing the success of reducing body fat mass, increasing fat-free mass, reducing waist circumference size, reducing BMI, and increasing body balance. These studies also successfully recorded immunoglobulin concentrations in saliva, testosterone levels, and the ability to perform ordered tasks [65]. The increments of salivary IgA values are shown to help prevent respiratory infections [66].

Improvement in functional capacity is also achieved by increasing walking speed as well as the results of body balance tests. This is in line with the addition of strength to the leg muscles [67]. An encouraging result was obtained, that by doing exercise, the subjects gained the effect of meaningful thinking ability. That ability to think and act may not be able to achieve normal IQ value, but at least it adds value to short-term memory ability and vocabulary and improves the ability to act and problem-solving [68].

One obstacle that participants with an intellectual disability face is getting distracted easily. The duration of maintaining concentration is also shorter than that of people with normal IQ. This situation greatly affects their motivation to complete the exercise session. In order to produce the desired exercises and their effects, the coaching team must intervene directly to interact with the participants with IDs. Caregiver involvement, as well as family, is very important to provide motivation and real examples of doing these movements. A cheerful atmosphere can be prevented by tuning in to the spirit-boosting music. IDs will be encouraged if they are given the expectation of rewards and appreciation, even if the rewards are simple. The coaching team must always be creative to be able to make the exercises as interesting games for them. It should also be realized that most IDs have mood patterns that are easy to change drastically [64].

Stijn et al. reiterated that safety is the priority concern for this group. The equipment used for this exercise has to be safe and not pose any danger, both intentional and unintentional. Basic equipment that was originally used to complement and help IDs in exercise can turn into a dangerous weapon, without them knowing or planning. It is also necessary to avoid sophisticated equipment such as robots. Movements have to be as simple as possible for them to comprehend and do properly and correctly [64, 65]. A simple example that they apparently cannot do is the squatting movement with ball between the back and the wall. They also cannot perform bridge pose. However, some research and observations explain that there is one movement they like and 100% are willing to repeat, and it is the biceps curl movement. There are times when the IDs do not want to make the movements ordered, so it is appropriate that the coaching team accompanies them by providing examples of these movements and opening up good communication.

Some research and observations state that there are also groups that can use simple and harmless RT tools. For example, using a chest press device is considered easier than using a bench press [69].

RT Recommendations for IDs:

1. Frequency 3x/week, with AE, preceded as warm-up also at the same time cooling-down, such as easy cycling and walking.

2. Short duration to prevent boredom, 45 minutes to a maximum of 60 minutes.

3. It is best to do RT in groups. There is a team that provides direct examples, also the participation of caregivers and families plays a very important role.

4. Full music, by designing the exercise as a team game. Whenever possible, hold gifts as encouragement.

5. Be careful when using tools, especially heavy or robotic equipment, because it can be an injurious weapon even if it is accidental.

6. The movements must be repeated frequently and as carefully as possible so they can do the movements properly and correctly.

7. Exercise involving 6–7 main muscles.

8. Two to three sets with 6–10 reps to avoid boredom.

## 8. Practical recommendations of RT for COVID-19 survivors

The new virus known as COVID-19 had shaken the world violently, and WHO in 2020 established pandemic status against COVID-19. WHO recorded 98 million people infected with 2.2 million deaths. Until now, the world remains vigilant and continues to fight COVID-19. Even after recovering from COVID-19, many writings and clinicians stated that there were many functional and even psychological declines complained by survivors. Sequelae felt, such as persistent muscle pain, fatigue even with minimal activity, muscle weakness, and frequent choking, the point is that they feel that their fitness status has deteriorated when compared to before getting COVID-19 [70].

This general functional deterioration is likely due to muscle atrophy resulting from immobilization during COVID-19 infection, as well as from muscle necrosis. This general functional deterioration is likely due to muscle atrophy resulting from immobilization during COVID-19 infection, as well as from muscle necrosis. Activation of the virus causes oxidative stress that induces overproduction of proinflammatory cytokines, resulting in corrosive cells damaging the myocyte. This damage will be more detrimental to the elderly population [71–73]. This is understandable because physiologically, people above 50 years will experience decrements of muscle mass 5–10% of the existing muscle mass. This decrease in muscle mass will result in the decrease in the functional capacity of the survivors. It is also aggravated by the disruption or difficulty of sleeping due to COVID-19. It is reported that this functional decline will result in depression. This condition will further reduce capacity of the immune system [74, 75].

Could exercise be used as a mean to restore physical functionality and reduce the level of depression in COVID-19 survivors? Deschenes MR [76] stated that exercise can improve morphological adaptations, such as increasing the amount of protein responsible for muscle contractiles and increasing the number of mitochondria [76]. Exercise is also believed to increase the immune system when done with a trusted, staged and sustainable dose.

A systematic review uploaded in 2022 involved research from November 2020 to January 2021, examining exercises given to 286 subject survivors of COVID-19 aged 20 to 84 years. In this study, survivors were trained in AE and RT. The intervention was AE (such as stationary bikes, walking, steps, and treadmill running), carried with low intensity (40–60%) and limited to 30 minutes. Meanwhile, RT was carried out with an average intensity of 50–70% 1xRM, 2 to 3 sets, with an average of 8–12 reps. Pre- and post-exercise evaluations were carried out by assessing the outcome of isokinetic strength, isometric strength, maximal strength, functional capacity, 6MWT, TUG, and strength grip. Exercises were performed for 10 to 12 weeks. Interventions targeted the lower and upper body [71]. Subjective feelings must also be maintained so that fatigue does not occur, which will then reduce the immune system [77]. There needs to be a restriction on subjective feelings limited to a scale of 4–6 out of 10 on the Modified Borg scale. All studies conducted showed better performance and decreased anxiety levels, which aimed certainly to improve the quality of life [70].

Exercise intensity, volume (set and reps) of RT, as well as duration must be carefully observed, so that the prescription of exercise is based on the initial value of functional performance. Some studies show that high-intensity exercise for about 1.5 hours per session is not recommended, because fatigue will occur and lead to decrease in the immune system [78–80]. Keep in mind that COVID-19 is closely related to the immune system, so the physical medicine and rehabilitation team must remain aware of possibility of decline in the immune system induced by exercise. Betschart et al. [81] shared their experience and noted that three patients were unable to continue their exercise therapy due to repeated bouts of the same infection [81]. Davis et al. in 1997 conducted a study on the effects of physical exercise on susceptibility to respiratory infection by using a murine model. They gave three different treatments: no exercise, moderate short-term exercise (30 minutes), and prolonged exercise to voluntary fatigue (2.5–3.5 h). It turned out that the results of exercise that are too long will cause fatigue that can trigger a higher mortality rate (41%) compared to groups with no exercise and moderate short-term exercise. Deaths in a group with no exercise reached 19%, while those who did moderate short-term exercise were only 9% [82]. According to the analysis carried out by Siedlik et al. in 2016 [83], heavy and longer exercise (more than 1 hour) can induce a suppressive effect on lymphocyte proliferative responses, with moderate strength statistically analyzed [83]. Some authors, such as Udina et al. [84], stated that short training period of 10 days has shown significant physical performance progress. Survivors do RT exercises: 30–80% 1xRM and limiting subjective feelings 3 to 5 of the modified Borgs scale [84]. Likewise, Herman et al. [85] reported there was no death case or hospitalization case in doing AE with moderate intensity, followed by 20 reps of RT exercises [85].

From these researchers' experiences, it can be concluded that COVID-19 survivors can carry out the combined exercise of AE and RT with safe composition. The prescription consists of AE: 5 to 30 minutes with low to moderate intensity, plus RT: 1–2 sets, 8–10 reps at 30–80% 1xRM. This prescription is also proven to increase muscle mass, muscle strength, reduce tightness when doing activities, reduce fatigue during activities, increase independence and ultimately improve quality of life. We have to stay alert and remain responsible for supervising every exercise. These studies still have shortcomings, such as not including the severity level of COVID-19.

## Conflict of interest

The authors declare no conflict of interest.

## Author details

Endang Ernandini[1*] and William Giovanni Mulyanaga[2]

1 Rehabilitation Center of Ministry of Defense, Jakarta, Indonesia

2 Padjadjaran University, Bandung, Indonesia

*Address all correspondence to: ernandiniebeb@gmail.com

## References

[1] Riebe D. ACSM's Guidelines for Exercise Testing and Prescription. 10th Edit ed. Philadelphia: Wolters Kluwer; 2018

[2] Silverthorn DU, Hill D. Human Physiology: An Integrated Approach. 7th ed. London: Pearson Education; 2016

[3] González-Badillo JJ, Sánchez-Medina L, Ribas-Serna J, Rodríguez-Rosell D. Toward a new paradigm in resistance training by means of velocity monitoring: A critical and challenging narrative. Sports Medicine - Open. 2022;**8**(1):118

[4] Kraemer WJ, Ratamess NA. Fundamentals of resistance training: Progression and exercise prescription. Medicine & Science in Sports & Exercise. 2004;**36**(4):674-688

[5] Folland JP, Williams AG. Morphological and neurological contributions to increased strength. Sports Medicine. 2007;**37**(2):145-168

[6] Spiering BA, Kraemer WJ, Anderson JM, Armstrong LE, Nindl BC, Volek JS, et al. Resistance exercise biology. Sports Medicine. 2008;**38**(7):527-540

[7] Bird SP, Tarpenning KM, Marino FE. Designing resistance training Programmes to enhance muscular fitness. Sports Medicine. 2005;**35**(10):841-851

[8] Harries S, Lubans D, Callister R. Resistance training to improve power and sports performance in adolescent athletes: A systematic review and meta-analysis. Journal of Science and Medicine in Sport. 2012;**15**:S222

[9] Suchomel TJ, Nimphius S, Bellon CR, Stone MH. The importance of muscular strength: Training considerations. Sports Medicine. 2018;**48**(4):765-785

[10] DeWeese BH, Hornsby G, Stone M, Stone MH. The training process: Planning for strength–power training in track and field. Part 2: Practical and applied aspects. Journal of Sport and Health Science. 2015;**4**(4):318-324

[11] Hall EJ. Guyton and Hall Textbook of Medical Physiology. 13th ed. United States: Elsevier; 2016. pp. 1085-1096

[12] American Thoracic Society. American College of Chest Physicians. ATS/ ACCP statement on cardiopulmonary exercise testing. American Journal of Respiratory and Critical Care Medicine. 2003;**167**(2):211-277

[13] Saikat Sengupta SC, Palash Kumar MN, Amitava Rudra SG. Cardiopulmonary exercise testing: A review of techniques and applications. Journal of Anesthesia Clinic Research. 2013;**04**(07) [Internet] [cited 2022 Nov 8]. Available from: https://www.omicsonline.org/cardiopulmonary-exercise-testing-a-review-of-techniques-and-applications-2155-6148.1000340.php?aid=16280

[14] Pollock ML, Franklin BA, Balady GJ, Chaitman BL, Fleg JL, Fletcher B, et al. AHA science advisory. Resistance exercise in individuals with and without cardiovascular disease: Benefits, rationale, safety, and prescription: An advisory from the committee on exercise, rehabilitation, and prevention, council on clinical cardiology, American Heart Association; position paper endorsed by the American College of Sports Medicine. Circulation. 2000;**101**(7):828-833

[15] Sherwood L. Human Physiology: From Cells to Systems. 7th ed. Belmont,

CA: Brooks/Cole, Cengage Learning; 2010

[16] Gharahdaghi N, Phillips BE, Szewczyk NJ, Smith K, Wilkinson DJ, Atherton PJ. Links between testosterone, Oestrogen, and the growth hormone/insulin-like growth factor Axis and resistance exercise muscle adaptations. Frontiers in Physiology [Internet]. 2021;**11** [cited 2022 Nov 8]. Available from: https://www.frontiersin.org/articles/10.3389/fphys.2020.621226

[17] Hooper DR, Kraemer WJ, Focht BC, Volek JS, DuPont WH, Caldwell LK, et al. Endocrinological roles for testosterone in resistance exercise responses and adaptations. Sports Medicine. 2017;**47**(9):1709-1720

[18] Hansen S, Kvorning T, Kjær M, Sjøgaard G. The effect of short-term strength training on human skeletal muscle: The importance of physiologically elevated hormone levels. Scandinavian Journal of Medicine & Science in Sports. 2001;**11**(6):347-354

[19] Ahtiainen JP, Pakarinen A, Alen M, Kraemer WJ, Häkkinen K. Muscle hypertrophy, hormonal adaptations and strength development during strength training in strength-trained and untrained men. European Journal of Applied Physiology. 2003;**89**(6):555-563

[20] Hermansen K, Bengtsen M, Kjær M, Vestergaard P, Jørgensen JOL. Impact of GH administration on athletic performance in healthy young adults: A systematic review and meta-analysis of placebo-controlled trials. Growth Hormone & IGF Research. 2017;**34**:38-44

[21] McCall GE, Byrnes WC, Fleck SJ, Dickinson A, Kraemer WJ. Acute and chronic hormonal responses to resistance training designed to promote muscle hypertrophy. Canadian Journal of Applied Physiology. 1999;**24**(1):96-107

[22] Ogasawara R, Sato K, Higashida K, Nakazato K, Fujita S. Ursolic acid stimulates mTORC1 signaling after resistance exercise in rat skeletal muscle. American Journal of Physiology. Endocrinology and Metabolism. 2013;**305**(6):E760-E765

[23] Bjersing JL, Larsson A, Palstam A, Ernberg M, Bileviciute-Ljungar I, Löfgren M, et al. Benefits of resistance exercise in lean women with fibromyalgia: Involvement of IGF-1 and leptin. BMC Musculoskeletal Disorders. 2017;**18**:106

[24] Kido K, Ato S, Yokokawa T, Makanae Y, Sato K, Fujita S. Acute resistance exercise-induced IGF1 expression and subsequent GLUT4 translocation. Physiological Reports. 2016;**4**(16):e12907

[25] Westcott WL. Resistance training is medicine: Effects of strength training on health. Current Sports Medicine Reports. 2012;**11**(4):209-216

[26] Flack KD, Davy KP, Hulver MW, Winett RA, Frisard MI, Davy BM. Aging, resistance training, and diabetes prevention. Journal of Aging Research. 2010;**2011**:127315

[27] Frontera WR, Hughes VA, Fielding RA, Fiatarone MA, Evans WJ, Roubenoff R. Aging of skeletal muscle: A 12-yr longitudinal study. Journal of Applied Physiology (Bethesda, MD: 1985). 2000;**88**(4):1321-1326

[28] Marcell TJ. Review article: Sarcopenia: Causes, consequences, and preventions. The Journals of Gerontology Series A: Biological Sciences and Medical Sciences. 2003;**58**(10):M911-M916

[29] Nelson ME, Fiatarone MA, Morganti CM, Trice I, Greenberg RA, Evans WJ. Effects of high-intensity strength training on multiple risk factors for osteoporotic fractures: A randomized controlled trial. Journal of the American Medical Association. 1994;**272**(24):1909-1914

[30] Wolfe RR. The underappreciated role of muscle in health and disease. The American Journal of Clinical Nutrition. 2006;**84**(3):475-482. DOI: 10.1093/ajcn/84.3.475

[31] Campbell WW, Crim MC, Young VR, Evans WJ. Increased energy requirements and changes in body composition with resistance training in older adults. The American Journal of Clinical Nutrition. 1994;**60**(2):167-175

[32] Hunter GR, Wetzstein CJ, Fields DA, Brown A, Bamman MM. Resistance training increases total energy expenditure and free-living physical activity in older adults. Journal of Applied Physiology. 2000;**89**(3):977-984

[33] Pratley R, Nicklas B, Rubin M, Miller J, Smith A, Smith M, et al. Strength training increases resting metabolic rate and norepinephrine levels in healthy 50- to 65-yr-old men. Journal of Applied Physiology. 1994;**76**(1):133-137

[34] Westcott WL, Winett RA, Annesi JJ, Wojcik JR, Anderson ES, Madden PJ. Prescribing physical activity: Applying the ACSM protocols for exercise type, intensity, and duration across 3 training frequencies. The Physician and Sportsmedicine. 2009;**37**(2):51-58

[35] Hunter GR, Bryan DR, Wetzstein CJ, Zuckerman PA, Bamman MM. Resistance training and intra-abdominal adipose tissue in older men and women. Medicine & Science in Sports & Exercise. 2002;**34**(6):1023-1028

[36] Treuth MS, Hunter GR, Kekes-Szabo T, Weinsier RL, Goran MI, Berland L. Reduction in intra-abdominal adipose tissue after strength training in older women. Journal of Applied Physiology. 1995;**78**(4):1425-1431

[37] Treuth MS, Ryan AS, Pratley RE, Rubin MA, Miller JP, Nicklas BJ, et al. Effects of strength training on total and regional body composition in older men. Journal of Applied Physiology. 1994;**77**(2):614-620

[38] Schmitz KH, Hannan PJ, Stovitz SD, Bryan CJ, Warren M, Jensen MD. Strength training and adiposity in premenopausal women: Strong, healthy, and empowered study. The American Journal of Clinical Nutrition. 2007;**86**(3):566-572

[39] Hurley BF, Hanson ED, Sheaff AK. Strength training as a countermeasure to aging muscle and chronic disease. Sports Medicine. 2011;**41**(4):289-306

[40] El-Kotob R, Ponzano M, Chaput JP, Janssen I, Kho ME, Poitras VJ, et al. Resistance training and health in adults: An overview of systematic reviews. Applied Physiology, Nutrition, and Metabolism. 2020;**45**(10 (Suppl. 2)):S165-S179

[41] Esco M. Resistance Training for Health and Fitness [Internet]. Philadelphia: American College of Sports Medicine; 2013. Available from: www.acsm.org

[42] Ernandini E, Pakasi TA, Santoso DIS, Tinduh D, Mirtha LT, Nasution SA, et al. Physical fitness assessment for lower limb disability: Rationale and design to develop a new formula. Bali Medical Journal. 2022;**11**(3):1262-1268

[43] Brellenthin AG, Lee D, chul, Bennie JA, Sui X, Blair SN. Resistance exercise, alone and in combination with aerobic exercise, and obesity in Dallas, Texas, US: A prospective cohort study. PLoS Medicine. 2021;**18**(6):e1003687

[44] Benefits of Modest Weight Loss in Improving Cardiovascular Risk Factors in Overweight and Obese Individuals with Type 2 Diabetes - PubMed [Internet]. [cited 2022 Nov 21]. Available from: https://pubmed.ncbi.nlm.nih.gov/21593294/

[45] Ryan DH, Yockey SR. Weight loss and improvement in comorbidity: Differences at 5%, 10%, 15%, and over. Current Obesity Reports. 2017;**6**(2):187-194

[46] Obesity [Internet]. [cited 2022 Nov 25]. Available from: https://www.who.int/westernpacific/health-topics/obesity

[47] Waist Circumference and Waist-Hip Ratio: Report of a WHO Expert Consultation [Internet]. [cited 2022 Nov 25]. Available from: https://www.who.int/publications-detail-redirect/9789241501491

[48] Jackson AW, Lee DC, Sui X, Morrow JR, Church TS, Maslow AL, et al. Muscular strength is inversely related to prevalence and incidence of obesity in adult men. Obesity (Silver Spring). 2010;**18**(10):1988-1995

[49] Lopez P, Taaffe DR, Galvão DA, Newton RU, Nonemacher ER, Wendt VM, et al. Resistance training effectiveness on body composition and body weight outcomes in individuals with overweight and obesity across the lifespan: A systematic review and meta-analysis. Obesity Reviews. 2022;**23**(5):e13428

[50] Liu X, Gao Y, Lu J, Ma Q, Shi Y, Liu J, et al. Effects of different resistance exercise forms on body composition and muscle strength in overweight and/or obese individuals: A systematic review and meta-analysis. Frontiers in Physiology. 2021;**12**:791999

[51] Stisen AB, Stougaard O, Langfort J, Helge JW, Sahlin K, Madsen K. Maximal fat oxidation rates in endurance trained and untrained women. European Journal of Applied Physiology. 2006;**98**(5):497-506

[52] Garrow JS, Summerbell CD. Meta-analysis: Effect of exercise, with or without dieting, on the body composition of overweight subjects. European Journal of Clinical Nutrition. 1995;**49**(1):1-10

[53] Sardeli AV, Komatsu TR, Mori MA, Gáspari AF, Chacon-Mikahil MPT. Resistance training prevents muscle loss induced by caloric restriction in obese elderly individuals: A systematic review and meta-analysis. Nutrients. 2018;**10**(4):423

[54] Cornelissen VA, Fagard RH, Coeckelberghs E, Vanhees L. Impact of resistance training on blood pressure and other cardiovascular risk factors. Hypertension. 2011;**58**(5):950-958

[55] Lewington S, Clarke R, Qizilbash N, Peto R, Collins R. Age-specific relevance of usual blood pressure to vascular mortality: A meta-analysis of individual data for one million adults in 61 prospective studies. Lancet. 2002;**360**(9349):1903-1913 [Internet]. [cited 2022 Nov 9] Available from: https://ora.ox.ac.uk/objects/uuid:d0e447ff-0440-4475-af76-d37c83a99da0

[56] Williams MA, Haskell WL, Ades PA, Amsterdam EA, Bittner V, Franklin BA, et al. Resistance exercise in individuals with and without cardiovascular

disease: 2007 update. Circulation. 2007;**116**(5):572-584

[57] Impact of Resistance Training on Arterial Stiffness [Internet]. Sci-Sport. [cited 2022 Nov 21]. Available from: https://www.sci-sport.com/en/articles/Impact-of-resistance-training-on-arterial-stiffness-209.php

[58] Haslam DRS, McCartney N, McKelvie RS, MacDougall JD. Direct measurements of arterial blood pressure during formal weightlifting in cardiac patients. Journal of Cardiopulmonary Rehabilitation and Prevention. 1988;**8**(6):213-225

[59] Wenger NK, Froelicher ES, Smith LK, Ades PA, Berra K, Blumenthal JA, et al. Cardiac rehabilitation as secondary prevention. Agency for Health Care Policy and Research and National Heart, Lung, and Blood Institute. Clinical Practice Guideline. Quick Reference Guide for Clinicians. 1995;**17**:1-23

[60] Kelemen MH. Resistive training safety and assessment guidelines for cardiac and coronary prone patients. Medicine and Science in Sports and Exercise. 1989;**21**(6):675-677

[61] Diagnostic and statistical manual of mental disorders: DSM-5™, 5th ed. Diagnostic and Statistical Manual of Mental Disorders: DSM-5™. 5th ed. Vol. xliv. Arlington, VA, US: American Psychiatric Publishing, Inc.; 2013. p. 947

[62] Dairo YM, Collett J, Dawes H, Oskrochi GR. Physical activity levels in adults with intellectual disabilities: A systematic review. Preventive Medical Reports. 2016;**4**:209-219

[63] Harris L, McGarty AM, Hilgenkamp T, Mitchell F, Melville CA. Correlates of objectively measured sedentary time in adults with intellectual disabilities. Preventive Medical Reports. 2018;**9**:12-17

[64] Weterings S, Oppewal A, van Eeden FMM, Hilgenkamp TIM. A resistance exercise set for a total body workout for adults with intellectual disabilities, a pilot study. Journal of Applied Research in Intellectual Disabilities. 2019;**32**(3):730-736

[65] Prescription and Effects of Strength Training in Individuals with Intellectual Disability—A Systematic Review - PMC [Internet]. [cited 2022 Nov 21]. Available from: https://www.ncbi.nlm.nih.gov/pmc/articles/PMC8470102/

[66] Chaushu S, Yefenof E, Becker A, Shapira J, Chaushu G. A link between parotid salivary Ig level and recurrent respiratory infections in young Down's syndrome patients. Oral Microbiology and Immunology. 2002;**17**(3):172-176

[67] Shields N, Taylor NF. A student-led progressive resistance training program increases lower limb muscle strength in adolescents with down syndrome: A randomised controlled trial. Journal of Physiotherapy. 2010;**56**(3):187-193

[68] Effects of Sixteen Week of Resistance Exercises on Some Selected Cognitive Variables Development in Adolescents with Intellectual Disabilities | Request PDF [Internet]. [cited 2022 Nov 21]. Available from: https://www.researchgate.net/publication/340280982_Effects_of_sixteen_week_of_resistance_exercises_on_some_selected_cognitive_variables_development_in_adolescents_with_intellectual_disabilities

[69] Iversen VM, Norum M, Schoenfeld BJ, Fimland MS. No time to lift? Designing time-efficient training programs for strength and hypertrophy:

A narrative review. Sports Medicine. 2021;**51**(10):2079-2095

[70] Ahmadi Hekmatikar AH, Ferreira Júnior JB, Shahrbanian S, Suzuki K. Functional and psychological changes after exercise training in post-COVID-19 patients discharged from the hospital: A PRISMA-compliant systematic review. International Journal of Environmental Research and Public Health. 2022;**19**(4):2290

[71] Alwardat N, Di Renzo L, de Miranda RC, Alwardat S, Sinibaldi Salimei P, De Lorenzo A. Association between hypertension and metabolic disorders among elderly patients in North Jordan. Diabetes & Metabolic Syndrome: Clinical Research & Reviews. 2018;**12**(5):661-666

[72] Pitscheider L, Karolyi M, Burkert FR, Helbok R, Wanschitz JV, Horlings C, et al. Muscle involvement in SARS-CoV-2 infection. European Journal of Neurology. 2021;**28**(10):3411-3417

[73] Jin M, Tong Q. Rhabdomyolysis as potential late complication associated with COVID-19. Emerging Infectious Diseases. 2020;**26**(7):1618-1620

[74] Gualtieri P, Falcone C, Romano L, Macheda S, Correale P, Arciello P, et al. Body composition findings by computed tomography in SARS-CoV-2 patients: Increased risk of muscle wasting in obesity. International Journal of Molecular Sciences. 2020;**21**(13):4670

[75] Saladino V, Algeri D, Auriemma V. The psychological and social impact of Covid-19: New perspectives of well-being. Frontiers in Psychology. 2020;**11**:577684

[76] Deschenes MR. Adaptations of the neuromuscular junction to exercise training. Current Opinion in Physiology. 2019;**10**:10-16

[77] Gentil P, de Lira CAB, Coswig V, Barroso WKS, PVO d V, Ramirez-Campillo R, et al. Practical recommendations relevant to the use of resistance training for COVID-19 survivors. Frontiers in Physiology. 2021;**12**:637590

[78] Suzuki K, Hayashida H. Effect of exercise intensity on cell-mediated immunity. Sports (Basel). 2021;**9**(1):8

[79] Gentil P, de Lira CAB, Souza D, Jimenez A, Mayo X, de Fátima Pinho Lins Gryschek AL, et al. Resistance training safety during and after the SARS-Cov-2 outbreak: Practical recommendations. BioMed Research International. 2020;**2020**:1-7

[80] Ferreira-Júnior JB, Freitas EDS, Chaves SFN. Exercise: A protective measure or an "open window" for COVID-19? A mini review. Frontiers in Sports and Active Living. 2020;**2** [Internet]. [cited 2022 Nov 20] Available from: https://www.frontiersin.org/articles/10.3389/fspor.2020.00061

[81] Betschart M, Rezek S, Unger I, Beyer S, Gisi D, Shannon H, et al. Feasibility of an outpatient training program after COVID-19. International Journal of Environmental Research and Public Health. 2021;**18**(8):3978

[82] Davis JM, Kohut ML, Colbert LH, Jackson DA, Ghaffar A, Mayer EP. Exercise, alveolar macrophage function, and susceptibility to respiratory infection. Journal of Applied Physiology. 1997;**83**(5):1461-1466

[83] Siedlik JA, Benedict SH, Landes EJ, Weir JP, Vardiman JP, Gallagher PM. Acute bouts of exercise induce a suppressive

effect on lymphocyte proliferation in human subjects: A meta-analysis. Brain, Behavior, and Immunity. 2016;**56**:343-351

[84] Udina C, Ars J, Morandi A, Vilaró J, Cáceres C, Inzitari M. Rehabilitation in adult post-COVID-19 patients in post-acute care with therapeutic exercise. The Journal of Frailty & Aging. 2021;**10**(3):297-300

[85] Hermann M, Pekacka-Egli AM, Witassck F, Baumgaertner R, Schoendorf S, Spielmanns M. Feasibility and efficacy of cardiopulmonary rehabilitation following COVID-19. American Journal of Physical Medicine & Rehabilitation. 2020;**99**(10):865-869. DOI: 10.1097/PHM.0000000000001549

Chapter 4

# Perspective Chapter: Resistance Exercises for Musculoskeletal Disorders

*Azzam Alarab and Nadeen Taqatqa*


## Abstract

Musculoskeletal disorders or MSDs are injuries and disorders that affect the human body's movement or musculoskeletal system (i.e. muscles, tendons, ligaments, nerves, discs, blood vessels, etc.). Popular musculoskeletal disorders is Carpal Tunnel Syndrome. Musculoskeletal fitness is integration of several aspect involve to unite mission of muscle strength, muscle endurance, and muscle power to showing power against one's own body weight or an external resistance.


**Keywords:** musculoskeletal disorders, resistance exercises, physiotherapy, manual therapy, strength exercises

## 1. Introduction

Musculoskeletal disorders, or MSDs, are impairment and damage that attack motion of the human body or the musculoskeletal system (such as muscles, tendons, ligaments, nerves, discs, blood vessels, etc.) Musculoskeletal diseases can be weaken hurt, its common health condition associated with aging Main symptoms are ache, hardness, inability to move easily and dexterity long period of time this conditions effect disability death rate and mental health [1]. One of the main causes of illness worldwide is musculoskeletal problems, which also have a significant detrimental effect on quality of life in terms of overall health. Other names for MSDs include "overuse injury," "repetitive motion injury," "repetitive stress injury," and several others. This terminology is links stress and repetition to a single factor that can harm the musculoskeletal system. This is limited because more and more research is pointing to multiple causative risk factors leading to MSDs [2].

Musculoskeletal disorders present a persistent and costly problem for society and contribute substantially to the global disease burden. The World Health Organization (WHO) reports that musculoskeletal disorders are the leading contributor to disablement globally in all sectors [3] at an estimated cost in 2019 of $13.11 billion USD [4].

Conditions affecting the musculoskeletal system include those that impact the joints, such as osteoarthritis, rheumatoid arthritis, psoriatic arthritis, gout, and spondyloarthritis; the bones, including such osteoporosis and associated fractures; the muscles, such as sarcopenia; and multiple physical areas or systems, such as regional (such as back and neck pain) and pervasive (such as fibromyalgia) pain conditions, inflammatory diseases such as connective tissue diseases and vasculitis that have musculoskeletal inflammatory diseases such as connective tissue diseases and vasculitis that have musculoskeletal manifestations, for example systemic lupus erythematosus, or amputation as a consequence of illness or trauma [5].

Musculoskeletal health is the result of a number of variables coming together. The joints and spine must be both solid and supple in order to support the body and perform a variety of activities to avid Arthritis and Rheumatism [6].

A healthy neurological system is necessary to regulate all of this activity, providing cohesion and balance, while strong muscles and solid bones are necessary to supply the strength to move. Additionally, excellent mental health is necessary to provide the drive and motivation to engage in physical activity. Additionally, this entire process should be completed "without pain, stiffness, or exhaustion" [7].

## 2. Musculoskeletal disorders causes

Muscles, tendons, ligaments, joints, and bones can all be impacted by musculoskeletal pain. A fracture, for example, might result in immediate, excruciating pain. Pain may also be brought on by a chronic illness like arthritis. Contact with a medical professional if your normal activities are hampered by musculoskeletal pain. The correct medical care can reduce your pain. Musculoskeletal pain has the potential to be acute, or abrupt and severe [8].

Or the discomfort can be ongoing (long-term). Pain could be restricted to one part of your body or could spread across it. They advise focusing on the following three major groups:

Painful musculoskeletal disorders including osteoarthritis and back pain are among the most prevalent. Lack of physical activity, weight, and injury are risk factors. Osteoporosis and fragility fractures, including inflammatory disorders like rheumatoid arthritis, affect 50% of women and 20% of men over the age of 50. This group of ailments is substantially less typical. The three main causes of musculoskeletal disorders are as follows:

High task repetition: Numerous work tasks and cycles are repetitive in nature and frequently under the management of work processes and hourly or daily output targets. When paired with other risk factors including high force and/or uncomfortable postures, high task repetition might contribute to the development of MSD. A job is considered highly repetitive if the cycle time is 30 seconds or less.

Forceful exertions: Many work tasks require high force loads on the human body. High force demands cause muscles to work harder, which raises associated fatigue and can cause MSD.

Awkward postures that are repeated or maintained put too much pressure on joints and overburden the muscles and tendons surrounding the affected joint.

Body joints function most effectively when they are most to their mid-range motion. When joints are operated outside of this mid-range repeatedly or for extended periods of time without enough healing time, the risk of MSD increases.

Musculoskeletal diseases can also be brought on by direct hits to the muscles, bones, or joints, such as one fractures, joint dislocations (when something pulls a joint away from its natural position), and sprains and strains [9].

Inflammatory Conditions: Arthritis Research UK describe "The Inflammatory Arthritis Pathway". It classifies inflammatory arthritis or autoimmune diseases as a group of conditions including rheumatoid arthritis, ankylosing spondylitis and psoriatic arthritis. The immune system attacks and destroys the joints and sometimes the internal organs. These relatively uncommon conditions affect less than one per cent of the population [6]. Evidence based guidelines such as the UK NICE Clinical Guideline for Rheumatoid Arthritis advocate specialist multidisciplinary input including pharmacological management. It also states that "people with RA should have access to specialist physiotherapy, with periodic review to improve general fitness and encourage regular exercise, and learn exercises for enhancing joint flexibility, muscle strength and managing other functional impairments" [10].

## 3. Overview of musculoskeletal conditions

Mechanical back pain: Often called back strain or musculoskeletal back pain. The etiology encompasses numerous causes, but the diagnosis excludes anatomical sources of pain such as a herniated disc or spondylosis. Common sources are strain of the paraspinal muscles (the muscles along the spine), strain of ligaments of the spine, or generative facet joint disease (the joints between the bones of the spine) [11].

Sciatica: This condition is usually caused by irritation of a nerve root of the sciatic nerve, often from compression by a disc or degenerative disease. Pain radiates into the buttocks, back of the thigh, and often into the calf or foot [12].

Radiculopathy: Dysfunction of the nerve root by any cause. Symptoms include weakness, pain (sciatica), numbness, paresthesias (tingling), or a combination thereof [13].

Herniated disc: Also called disc rupture, disc prolapse, or herniated nucleus pulposus (the gelatinous inner core of the disc). The annulus fibrosis is the outer layer of the disc, which is the strongest portion of the disc and provides the strength to prevent disc herniations. With age or injury, the wall of the spinal discs can become damaged and the wall of the disc can weaken and protrude. Disc pain is often felt as a deep ache in sacroiliac can be in the same location and feel the same [14].

Spinal Stenosis: This is a narrowing of the spinal canal, typically in the neck (cervical stenosis) or lower back (lumbar stenosis). The narrowing is called spondylosis. The etiology can vary (degenerative, trauma, congenital), but the most common spondylosis is a degenerative disorder, occurring with age. The hallmark of lumbar stenosis is pain in the back and legs that is aggravated by standing or walking and relieved by sitting or forward bending [15].

Myofascial pain: Refers to soft-tissue pain usually arising from trauma, repetitive activities, or poor posture. It is usually associated with muscle spasm. Patients may complain of pain in the neck region or pain across the top of the shoulders and sometimes sleep difficulties or headaches [16].

Scoliosis: This condition is an abnormal curvature of the spine. It has many causes, but the most common type is adolescent idiopathic scoliosis. Females are affected 8 times as frequently as males. In general, most forms of scoliosis are not specifically painful but may depend on the degree of curvature of the spine and/or the presence of degenerative spinal changes. Patients with a curvature.30 degrees may have more back pain during their lifetime than a person with a straight spine [17].

Fibromyalgia: Literally means muscle/soft-tissue pain. Patients complain of generalized myalgia, stiffness, or soreness. The pain is disseminated and occurs in different areas of the body at different times. The pain can increase with menstrual cycle or with sudden weather changes. A key diagnostic feature is concurrent fatigue and sleep disorder, with disruption of stage 4 sleep (an alpha EEG anomaly). Pain appears to improve with medications, physical exercise, and efforts to promote normal sleep patterns. Patients may have neurological disturbances such as headaches, numbness, weakness, difficulty concentrating, and lightheadedness. As many as 50% of patients have clinical depression in their lifetime [18].

## 4. Clinical features for musculoskeletal disorders

Symptoms of musculoskeletal illnesses might vary. One of the initial symptoms is chronic pain, albeit how it manifests itself differs from person to person. Some people experience pain throughout their bodies, while others may just pain occurs in a specific area. The typical symptoms are:

- Aching & stiffness joints.
- Pain that worsens with movement.
- Difficulty in moving.
- Fatigue.
- Inflammation.
- Tenderness.
- Swelling.
- Muscle spasm.
- Bruising and discoloration.
- Warmth.

Depending on the type of MSD that has occurred, different symptoms will appear. For instance, osteoarthritis results in stiff, tight joints and painful, spasm of muscles [19, 20].

## 5. Medical treatment for musculoskeletal disorders

Musculoskeletal pain is a serious medical issue in both its acute and chronic forms.

The problem is widespread in primary care settings, and it set of assets for the majority of people who visit pain clinics. The problem typically manifests as neck and back discomfort. However, it is typically impossible to provide a pathoanatomic diagnosis of the origin of pain. The majority of musculoskeletal pain problems are therefore classified anatomically as regional pain syndromes, including neck and back pain. Standard diagnostic labels for shoulder pain include frozen shoulder, subacromial bursitis, supraspinatus tendinitis, and many others. However, recent research has revealed that these disorders cannot be reliably or validly diagnosed using the traditional diagnostic methods [4–6]. As a result, even shoulder pain is classified as a local musculoskeletal disorder Knee pain may result from injuries to the menisci or other intra-articular structures [21].

## 6. Evidence based practice for musculoskeletal disorders

There have been a few paradigm shifts in the field of physiotherapy and its practice as a result of EBP or scientific study.

Among them are the following:

1. Bed rest for back pain: Although bed rest has long been prescribed for back pain, its therapeutic value has just recently been examined. The most typical course of treatment for back pain and sciatica is to recommend rest, give analgesics, and treat acute bouts with bed rest. Although this advice is supported by orthopedic instruction, there are growing reservations and dissatisfactions about this kind of management [22]. Both important studies by Gilbert et al. and Deyo et al. demonstrated that longer periods of bed rest offer no advantages over shorter ones. The 1994 clinical guidelines suggest activity restriction and urge short, 2–4 day periods of bed rest [19]. Even brief intervals of relaxation have come under scrutiny more lately. Despite trying to produce a number of negative side effects as joint stiffness, muscle atrophy, loss of bone mineral density, pressure sores, and venous thromboembolism, bed rest did not significantly alleviate symptoms compared to other treatments [23].

2. Early Mobilization in Intensive Care setting: Early Mobilization in the Intensive Care Setting Attempts at full active mobilization are frequently postponed until the acute stage of the illness has passed. In particular, it is recognized that rehabilitation may not begin until after ICU discharge, that's because the patients are thought to be too ill to engage while undergoing mechanical breathing. These traditional practices are only the result of expert opinion and are not supported by solid research [24]. After conducting a systematic review of the literature on the impact of early mobilization, ***Joseph Adler and Daniel Malone (2012) came to the conclusion that physical therapy and early mobilization are both safe and effective interventions that can significantly improve patient symptoms and functional outcomes like muscle strength and functional mobility [25].

## 7. Physiotherapy protocol for musculoskeletal disorders

### 7.1 Joint protection/fatigue management

There is strong support for the claim that, when given as a behavioral group program, this lessens pain, early morning stiffness, maintains functional capacity, improves grip, and decreases the number of visits to a doctor for arthritis one year after receiving information about early RA [26].

### 7.2 Assistive devices

The use of assistive technology eases discomfort and makes daily chores easier (ADL). Nationwide, the availability is uneven (**Figure 1**) [27, 28].

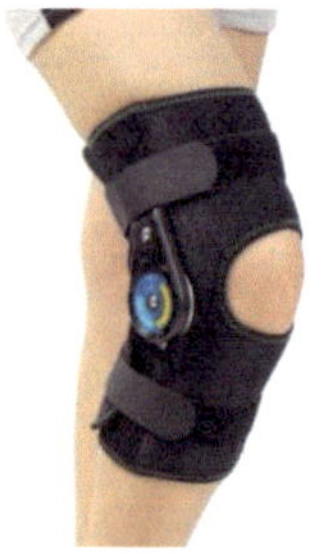

**Figure 1.**
*Assistive device, ACL brace with range of motion [29].*

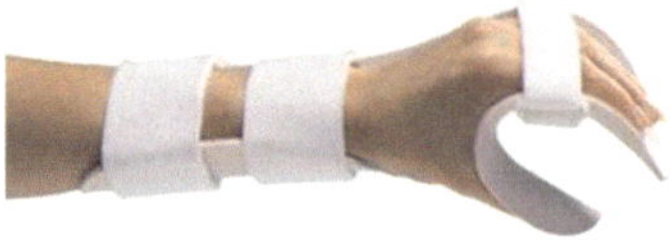

**Figure 2.**
*Hand splinting, Cocup Splint [32].*

## 7.3 Hand splinting

When worn, wrist splints lessen discomfort and enhance functionality.

Pain is lessened at night by resting splints [30]. There is currently no proof that splinting prevents deformity or long-term function maintenance. To ensure the most therapeutic benefit, staff who have been trained in their usage must accurately fit all splints, fully explain how to use them, and regularly review them (**Figure 2**) [31].

## 7.4 Exercises

1. For up to a year, comprehensive physiotherapy (education, exercise, and pain management modalities) reduces early morning stiffness [33–35].

2. Aerobic and strengthening exercise. Two systematic reviews conclude this leads to significant improvements in physical (muscle strength, aerobic capacity, endurance and function) and psychological status (self-efficacy and well-being) and does not exacerbate disease activity [36, 37]**.** People with arthritis should be taught an efficient exercise regimen that combines moderate strength training (50–80% of maximal voluntary contraction) twice to three times per week with moderate aerobic exercise (60–85% of maximum heart rate) three times per week for a total of 30 to 60 minutes.

3. Exercise on Prescription' schemes (i.e. free/reduced rate exercise facilities available in leisure centres following referral by a GP for health reasons) should also be available for people with arthritis.

4. Hand exercise (provided by both Occupational Therapist and Physiotherapist). For enhancing grip and pinch strength, reducing discomfort, and maintaining hand function, range of motion and strength exercises work better together than either range of motion or wax therapy alone (**Figures 3–6**) [33].

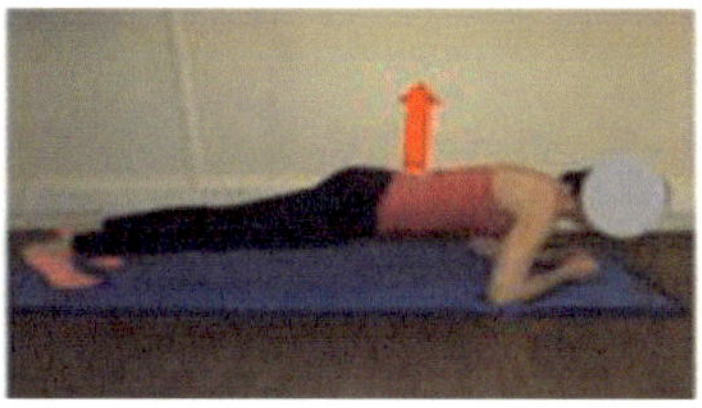

**Figure 3.**
*Strengthening exercise for trunk stabilization [38].*

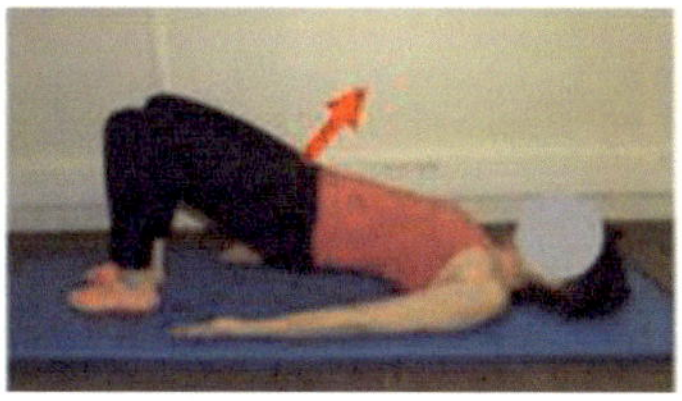

**Figure 4.**
*Strengthening exercise for gluteus muscles [38].*

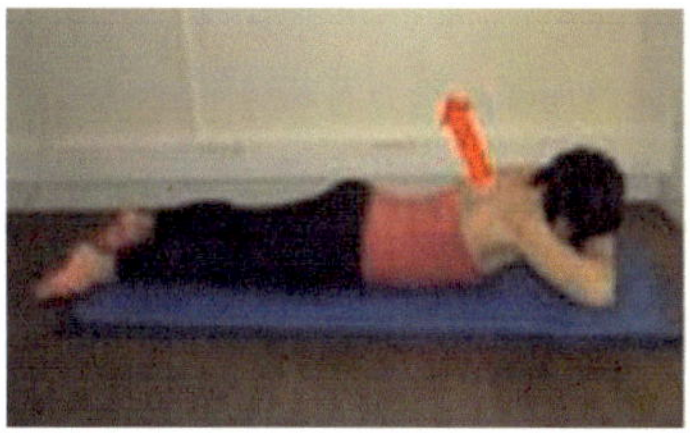

**Figure 5.**
*Strengthening exercise for back muscles [38].*

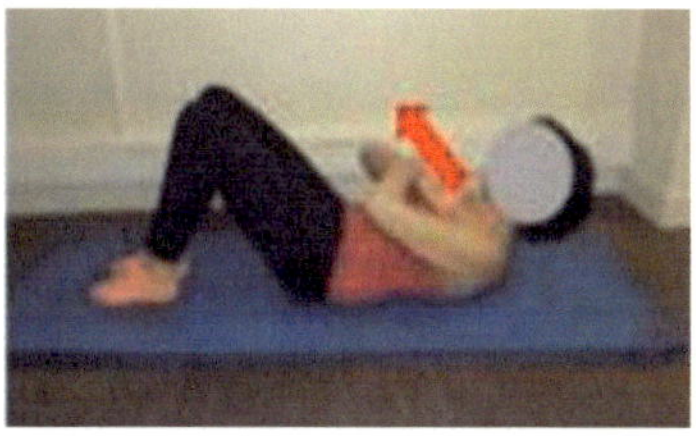

**Figure 6.**
*Strengthening exercise for abdominal muscles [38].*

### 7.5 Hydrotherapy

There is some indication that by maintaining activity levels, hospitalizations are not as necessary.

It costs a lot of money and is not widely available (**Figure 7**) [39].

### 7.6 Thermotherapy

Apart from temporary symptom relief, using heat and ice packs, using cryotherapy, or taking faradic baths does not have any substantial advantages.

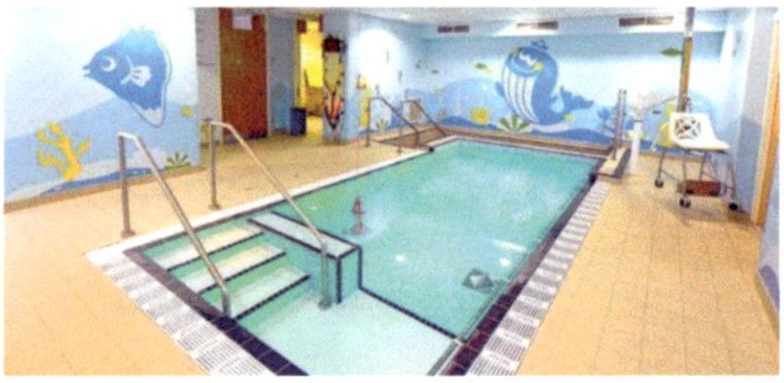

**Figure 7.**
*Hydrotherapy [40].*

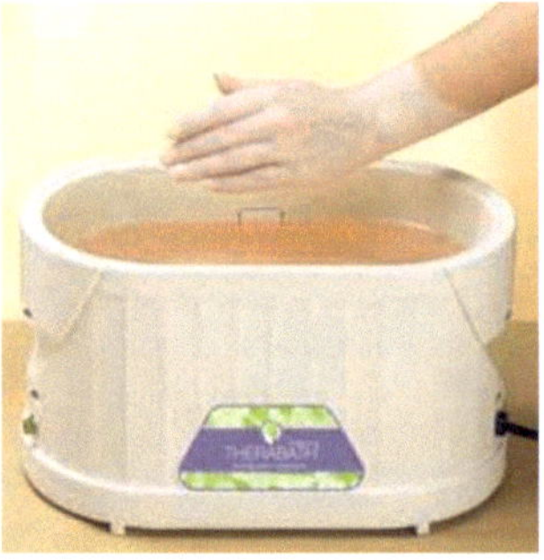

**Figure 8.**
*Thermotherapy, paraffin wax [42].*

Exercises and paraffin wax baths offer positive short-term effects for arthritic hands (**Figure 8**) [33, 41].

### 7.7 Electrical stimulation

Increases muscle strength and endurance training for patients who are unable to properly activate their muscles on their own. Only one short, high-quality study, however, has demonstrated how ES improves hand grip strength and fatigue resistance (**Figure 9**) [43].

### 7.8 Low level laser therapy and acupuncture

These have no other impacts other helping to quickly lessen pain. However, there aren't many small-scale trials (**Figures 10** and **11**) [45, 46].

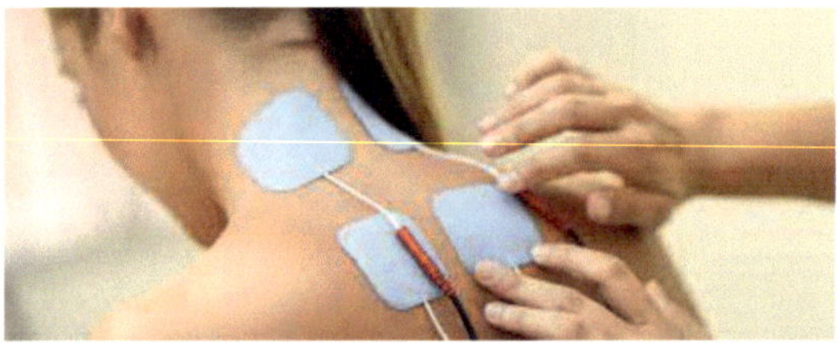

**Figure 9.**
*Electrical stimulation [44].*

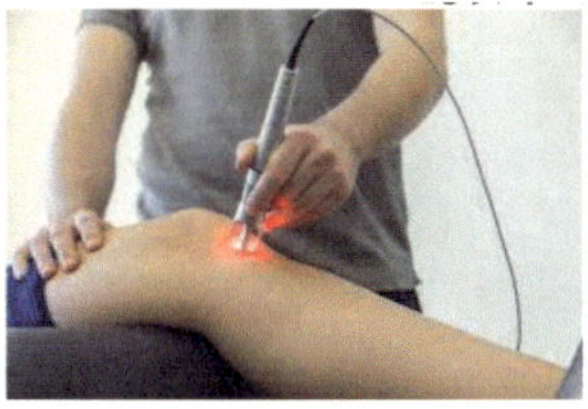

**Figure 10.**
*Laser therapy [47].*

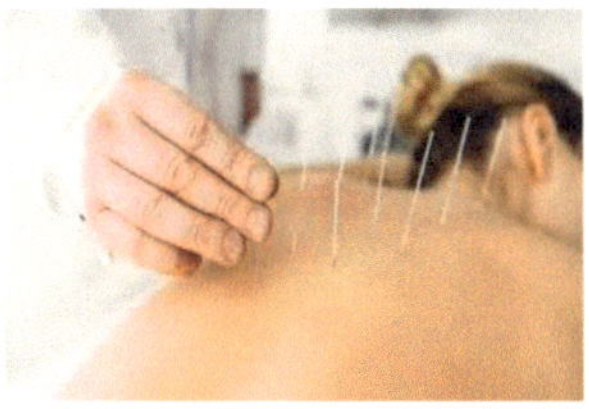

**Figure 11.**
*Acupuncture [48].*

### 7.9 Multidisciplinary rehabilitation

For those with active RA or moderate-severe RA and various functional issues, coordinated intense multidisciplinary rehabilitation programs are crucial. Both in-patient rehabilitation and intensive medical care delivered in well-organized, coordinated day care are advantageous, with day care being marginally less expensive.

The most efficient way to deliver multidisciplinary care for patients with more severe difficulties is probably influenced by local geography and service characteristics [49–51].

## 8. Therapeutic agents for musculoskeletal disorders

The use of thermal, mechanical, electromagnetic, and light energy for therapeutic reasons is referred to as therapeutic modalities [52]. Physiotherapists frequently use these to assist their patients' or clients' therapy goals:

- Reduction or modification of pain
- Reduce inflammation,
- Enhance circulation,
- Promote tissue healing,
- Restructure scar tissue.
- Treatment for skin issues,
- An increase in range of motion,

- and improved muscular activation.
- Reduced or eliminated oedema,
- preservation of strength following injury or surgery, and reduction edema [53, 54].

For many years, physiotherapy has made use of therapeutic methods. Although there is some evidence that different patients may benefit from different modalities, it is suggested that they should not be used as a stand-alone treatment. Instead, they are frequently used in conjunction with other physiotherapy tools, such as exercise, manual techniques, and patient education [55, 56].

To refer to all therapies that have physiological therapeutic effects, the phrases "therapeutic modalities" and "electrophysical agents" are frequently mixed [52].

Therapeutic techniques include, for instance:

- Electrical stimulation/Iontophoresis.
- Biofeedback.
- Thermotherapy (superficial or deep).
- Cryotherapy.
- Ultrasound/Phonophoresis.
- Extracorporeal Shockwave Therapy (ESWT).
- Laser therapy.
- Magnetic therapy.
- Massage.
- Mechanical traction.

According to different grades of evidence, clinical guidelines support the use of therapeutic modalities [57].

However, the decision regarding which modality to use may be influenced by the patient's requirements and goals, the clinician's preferences, and the condition at hand [58].

## 9. Manual therapy for musculoskeletal disorders

Physical therapists have made significant achievements to the current diversity in manual therapy approaches and procedures. Manual therapy has a lengthy history within the physical therapy profession. In the past, mechanical justifications were employed to describe how manual therapy techniques functioned. Intricate neurophysiologic mechanisms are also at work, according to recent study, and offering hands-on assessment and intervention has been shown to have positive psychological impacts [59].

- Physiological: positive placebo response.
- Biomechanical and physical: facilitates repair and tissue modeling
- Psychological benefits include pain alleviation by stimulation of the gating mechanism, muscular inhibition, a decrease in nociceptive activity, and a reduction in intraarticular or periarticular pressure [60].

### 9.1 Manual therapy frameworks: Maitland manual therapy

System of Prescription: Joints, muscles and nervous tissue in both the spine and peripheral joints. Area: Observing the symptoms and using the most effective therapy strategy are more crucial than figuring out the root cause of the dysfunction right away:

Additionally seeks to resolve a specific functional issue by eradicating discomfort, regaining joint mobility, and restoring normal muscle tension. Treatment Methods: Rhythmic, passive, painless movements introduced into the tissue (mobilizations) and rapid movements (manipulations) (**Figure 12**).

### 9.2 McKenzie manual therapy

System of Prescription: Spine-healing therapy utilizing patient movement that is active, supported by movement, and passive.

Area: Spine.

Treatment Approaches: The patient and the therapist are searching for a movement pattern that, after a few repetitions, shows a meaningful improvement (**Figure 13**).

### 9.3 Mulligan manual therapy

System of Prescription: Mulligan's therapy is based on patient movement that is both active and passively corrected by the physiotherapist holding the joint.

Area: Spine and limbs, with a focus on disorders that impact the periphery.

Methods of treatment:

- Pain free, effective compression of the articular surfaces with gravity.
- Active movement combined with passive movement in the plane of the articular surfaces.

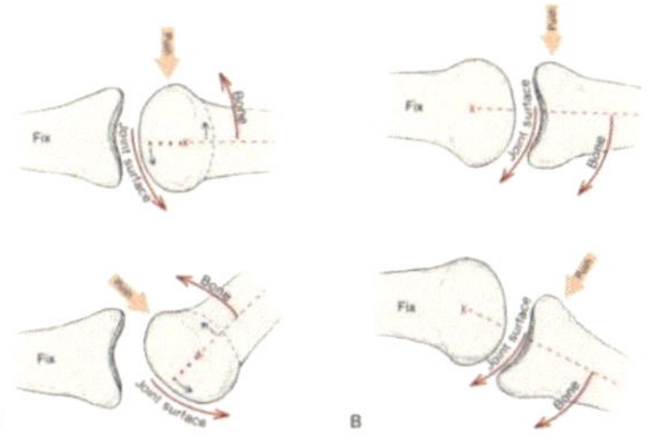


**Figure 12.**
*Convex-Concave Rule for Maitland Mobilization [61].*

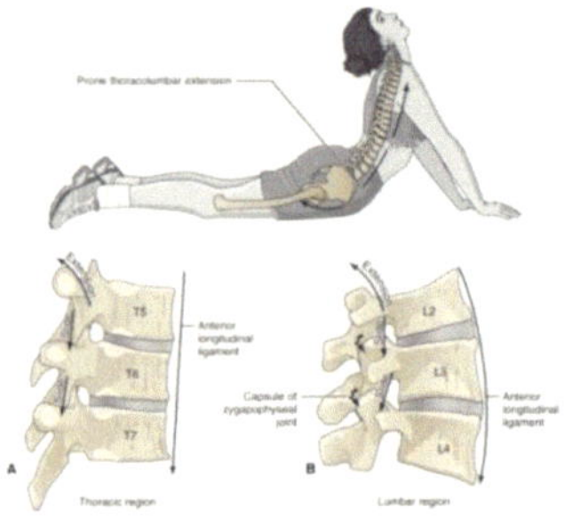

**Figure 13.**
*McKenzie extension exercise [62].*

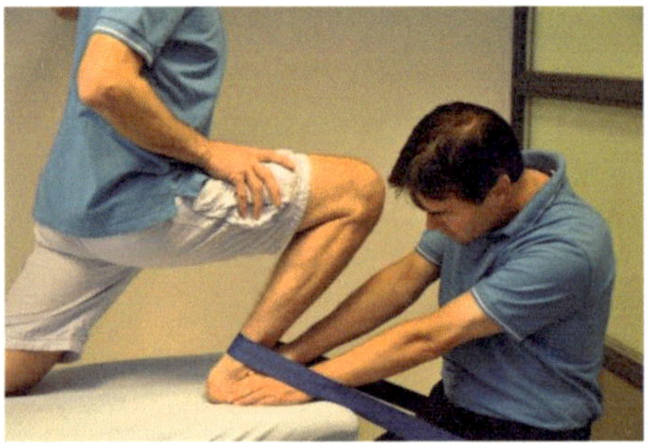

**Figure 14.**
*Mulligan Technique (MWMS) [64].*

- Applying an acceptable number of repetitions.
- Applying overpressure at the limit of the pleasant movement range (**Figure 14**) [63].

## 10. Hydrotherapy for musculoskeletal disorders

Any activity done in the water to aid in healing and rehabilitation after a strenuous workout or significant injury is referred to as hydrotherapy (Aquatherapy) [65, 66]. It is a common method of treatment for people with musculoskeletal and neurologic disorders and involves activity in warm water [67]. Muscle relaxation, increased joint motion, and pain relief are the aims of this therapy [68]. This therapy is been used for thousands of years.

### 10.1 Physiological effects

The physiological outcomes of water therapy bring together the advantages of the exercises and the heated pool water. The duration of the treatment, the water's temperature, the type and intensity of the activity, and the magnitude of the effects all vary [69]. Exercise in the water has physiological consequences that are similar to those of exercise on land. With each chemical shift that takes place while the muscles contract, more blood is supplied to the active muscles, which in turn causes the muscles' temperature to rise. The muscles have a higher metabolic rate, which causes a higher demand for oxygen and a higher output of carbon dioxide. This impact is a result of both these modifications and the equivalent modifications caused by the water's heat. Muscle power improves while the amount of joint motion is either maintained or expanded. The physiological effects of the soaking are less localized than those caused by any other source of heat. Since the body absorbs heat from the water and from all the contracting muscles used during activity, a rise in body temperature is unavoidable. The superficial blood vessels expand as the skin warms up, increasing the peripheral blood flow. By means of convection, the temperature of the underlying tissues rises as a result of the heated blood flowing through these capillaries [70].

### 10.2 Therapeutic effects

- Relieve pain and muscle spasm.
- To gain relaxation.
- To maintain or increase the range of joint movement.
- To re-educate paralyzed muscles.
- To strengthen weak muscles and to develop their power and endurance.
- To encourage walking and other functional and recreational activities.
- To increase blood flow (trophic condition of the skin).
- To boost the patient's morale by encouraging and reassuring him to perform his workouts [69, 70].
- By acting on temperature receptors and mechanoreceptors, the warmth of water inhibits nociception and affects spinal segmental processes [67].

## 11. Resistance exercises for musculoskeletal disorder

Muscles are forced to operate against a weight or force during strength training, commonly referred to as resistance exercise. Resistance exercise is an anaerobic exercise [71]. The use of free weights, weight machines, resistance bands, and your own body weight are a few examples of various forms of strength training. For the most benefit, a beginner should exercise two to three times each week. Before beginning a new

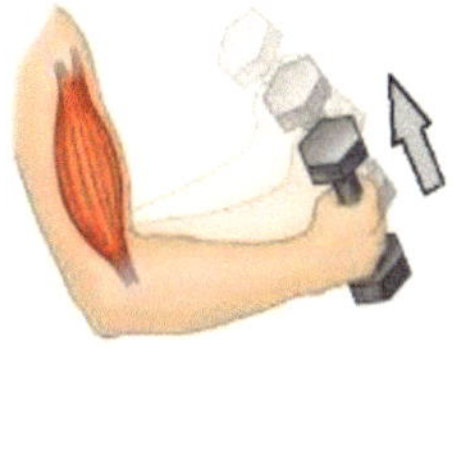

**Figure 15.**
*Isotonic exercise [73].*

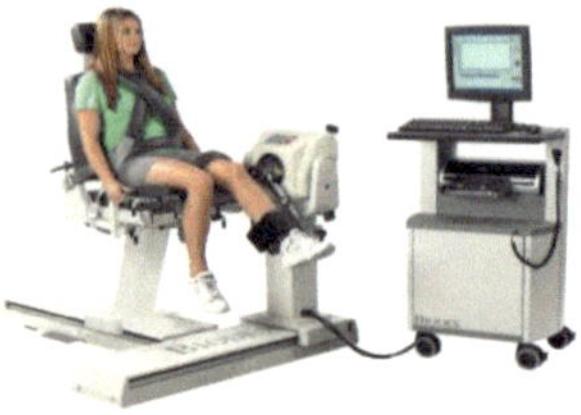

**Figure 16.**
*Isokinetic exercise [74].*

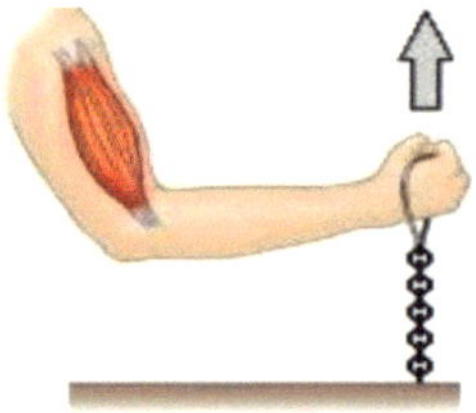

**Figure 17.**
*Isometric exercise [73].*

fitness program, the patient should undergo a pre-participation health examination and contact with professionals such as a doctor, exercise physiologist, physiotherapist, or licensed exercise professional. To enhance strength and growth increases, players should rest each muscle group for at least 48 hours. Vary workouts to help client push past a training plateau [72]. Comes in three forms: isotonic, isometric, and isokinetic.

- Isotonic consists of dynamic movements with a constant load (**Figure 12**).
- Isokinetic involves a constant velocity with variable load (**Figure 13**).
- Isometric involves muscle contraction that is static with no change in muscle length (**Figures 15–17**) [75].

## 12. Effects of strength training

Numerous advantageous neuromuscular changes that improve both physical and mental health are promoted by strength training.

Resistance exercise has several advantages for both mental and physical health, including:

- increased muscle tone and strength.
- Keeping your balance, mobility, and flexibility can let you age independently.
- Weight management and a higher muscle-to-fat ratio may be even more helpful for fat loss than aerobic exercise [71].
- Could aid in slowing or stopping cognitive decline in older persons.

- Greater stamina: You will not tire as easily as you do when you get stronger.
- avoidance or management of chronic illnesses like obesity, diabetes, depression, arthritis, vascular disease, and back pain.
- Pain relief,
- better posture
- lower risk of injury.
- increased bone strength and density, as well as a decreased chance of osteoporosis.
- Increased feeling of wellness — resistance training may improve mood, body image, and self-esteem.
- Better sleep and a reduction in insomnia.
- Improved blood lipid profiles
- reduced resting blood pressure
- increased gastrointestinal transit speed
- increased blood glucose utilization [72].

## 13. Comparison between resistance exercises and physical therapy

Strength training improves your capacity to overcome resistance by having you concentrate on lifting the most weight for the specified amount of repetitions. Physical therapy programs for the treatment of a variety of musculoskeletal problems always incorporate strength training. Moving the weight from point A to point B is the main concern [76]. With stronger muscles, almost every action becomes easier. Exercise treatment may provide benefits to patients with chronic low back pain through the voluntary contraction of specific muscle groups [77, 78].

## 14. International modern studies about treatment for musculoskeletal disorders

Musculoskeletal Disorders and Treatment focus on various aspects of Repetitive Motion Injuries, Repetitive Strain Injuries, Cumulative Trauma Disorders, Occupational Cervicobrachial Disorders, Overuse Syndrome, Regional Musculoskeletal Disorders, Soft Tissue Disorders, Work-Related Musculoskeletal Disorders, Musculoskeletal Disorders in the Elderly, Arthritis, Drug Interaction Checker, Fibromyalgia, Living Healthy, Lupus Osteoarthritis, Pill Identifier, Rheumatoid Arthritis, Sports Injuries, etc. Original Article, Reviews, Mini Reviews, Short Communications, Case Reports, Clinical Image, Perspectives/Opinions, Letters, Short Note and Commentaries are acceptable for publication [79].

### 14.1 Pain reduction

One trial with 40 individuals that produced very low quality data demonstrated a clinically significant advantage of exercise over standard therapy after around three months.

9 studies with 528 people produced very bad quality evidence that at >3 months, there was no clinically significant difference between exercise and conventional treatment. At >3 months, there was no clinically significant difference between exercise and usual care, according to very low quality evidence from 1 study with 95 participants.

### 14.2 Health related quality of life

Five studies with 372 participants and very low quality data each shown a clinically significant advantage of exercise over standard therapy after >3 months. One study with 54 participants found very low to low quality evidence that exercise had a clinically significant advantage over standard care after more than three months. Regular care was found to have a clinically significant advantage compared to exercise at about three months in one study with 95 individuals using very low to low quality data. 259 people in 2 studies with very low quality evidence demonstrated a clinically significant advantage of exercise compared to conventional treatment at >3 months. Very low quality evidence from 1 study 95 participants showed no clinically important difference between exercise and usual care at ≤3 months or at >3 months.

### 14.3 Physical function

Very low quality data from 2 studies with 155 people and 1 research with 95 participants indicated no clinically relevant difference between exercise and usual care at 3 months and no clinically important difference between exercise and usual care at >3 months, respectively.

Three studies with 169 participants and very low quality data each shown a clinically significant advantage of exercise over standard care after more than three months. Three studies with a total of 246 individuals produced very low quality evidence that exercise had a clinically significant advantage over standard care after more than three months.

### 14.4 Psychological distress

One trial with 60 individuals produced low quality evidence that exercise had a clinically significant advantage over standard therapy after about three months. A lack of clinically significant differences between exercise and usual care at >3 months was revealed by low quality data from 3 studies with 123 participants. At >3 months, there was no clinically significant difference between exercise and standard care, according to low quality data from 4 studies with 306 individuals. At >3 months, there was no clinically significant difference between exercise and standard care, according to low quality data from 4 studies with 320 participants. One trial with 50 individuals that had very low quality data found no clinically significant difference between usual treatment and exercise after more than three months. There was no clinically significant difference between exercise and standard treatment after >3 months, according to very low quality data from 1 research with 95 individuals [80].

## 15. Conclusion

Physical activity and exercise are crucial components of a healthy lifestyle. Exercises associated with daily living such as walking, housework and gardening can be enhanced with activities that are typically regarded exercise, such as sports activities and joining a gym. Enhancing physical exercise is frequently advised for those who suffer from chronic pain. Determining the sort and volume of exercise that would lessen the burden of pain on their lives, develop healthy exercise habits, and allow them to benefit from the wider range of health effects of leading an active lifestyle presents a problem for persons with pain. For those who are in discomfort, keeping the urge to keep working out could be more challenging. Exercises that increase the strength of particular muscles or muscle groups are known as strengthening exercises. The force and muscular overload promote growth and boost power. Weak muscles can increase the risk of injury to the joints and surrounding soft tissues. Patients with muscle illnesses are offered strengthening exercises as part of their treatment regimen since they are an essential component of physical therapy.

## Acknowledgements

I thank the student, Nadeen Taqatqa, for her contribution and assistance in completing this project.

## Conflict of interest

The authors declare no conflict of interest.

## Abbreviations

| | |
|---|---|
| MSDs | musculoskeletal disorders |
| EBP | evidence based practice |
| RA | rheumatoid arthritis (RA) |
| ADL | activity daily life |
| GP | general practitioner |
| ES | electrical stimulation |
| ESWT | extracorporeal shock-wave therapy |
| MWMS | mobilization with movements |

## Author details

Azzam Alarab* and Nadeen Taqatqa
Faculty of Allied Medical Sciences, Physiotherapy Department, Palestine Ahliya University, Bethlehem, Palestine

*Address all correspondence to: nadeen.taqatqa15@gmail.com

## References

[1] GBD Cirrhosis Collaborators. The global, regional, and national burden of cirrhosis by cause in 195 countries and territories, 1990-2017: A systematic analysis for the Global Burden of Disease Study 2017. Lancet Gastroenterology and Hepatology. 2020;**5**(3):245-266. DOI: 10.1016/S2468-1253(19)30349-8

[2] Liao CD, Chen HC, Huang SW, Liou TH. The role of muscle mass gain following protein supplementation plus exercise therapy in older adults with sarcopenia and frailty risks: A Systematic Review and Meta-Regression Analysis of Randomized Trials. Nutrients. 2019;**11**(8):1713. DOI: 10.3390/nu11081713

[3] WHO. Musculoskeletal Conditions. 2019. Available from: https://www.who.int/news-room/factsheets/detail/musculoskeletal-conditions

[4] Liberty Mutual. 2019 Liberty Mutual Workplace Safety Index. 2019. Available from: https://business.libertymutualgroup.com/business-insurance/Documents/Services/DS200.pdf

[5] Cieza A, Causey K, Kamenov K, Hanson SW, Chatterji S, Vos T. Global estimates of the need for rehabilitation based on the Global Burden of Disease study 2019: A systematic analysis for the Global Burden of Disease Study 2019. Lancet. 2021;**396**(10267):2006-2017. DOI: 10.1016/S0140-6736(20)32340-0

[6] Sammaritano LR, Bermas BL, Chakravarty EE, et al. 2020 American College of Rheumatology Guideline for the management of reproductive health in rheumatic and musculoskeletal diseases. Arthritis & Rhematology. 2020;**72**(4):529-556. DOI: 10.1002/art.41191

[7] Smith BE, Hendrick P, Bateman M, et al. Musculoskeletal pain and exercise-challenging existing paradigms and introducing new. British Journal of Sports Medicine. 2019;**53**(14):907-912. DOI: 10.1136/bjsports-2017-098983

[8] Arthritis Research UK. Policy and Public Health document.

[9] Akazawa N, Okawa N, Kishi M, Hino T, Tsuji R, Tamura K, et al. Quantitative features of intramuscular adipose tissue of the quadriceps and their association with gait independence in older inpatients: A cross-sectional study. Nutrition. 2020;**71**:110600. DOI: 10.1016/j.nut.2019.110600

[10] Arthritis Research UK. Policy and Public Health document

[11] National Institute for Health and Care Excellence (NICE). Low back pain and sciatica in over 16s: Assessment and management. 2020

[12] NCD Risk Factor Collaboration (NCD-RisC). Heterogeneous contributions of change in population distribution of body mass index to change in obesity and underweight. Elife. 2021;**10**:e60060. DOI: 10.7554/eLife.60060

[13] Park JS, Yoo JI, Na JB, Song HS. The prevalence and risk factors of musculoskeletal disorders in the hands of fishermen working as oyster shuckers. International Journal of Occupational Medical Environmental Health. 2021;**34**(5):603-615. DOI: 10.13075/ijomeh.1896.01752

[14] Will JS, Bury DC, Miller JA. Mechanical low back pain. American Family Physician. 2018;**98**(7):421-428

[15] Jensen RK, Kongsted A, Kjaer P, Koes B. Diagnosis and treatment of sciatica. BMJ. 2019;**367**:l6273. DOI: 10.1136/bmj.l6273

[16] Carnevale JA, Goldberg JL, Schwarz J. Lumbar herniated disc. World Neurosurgery. 2022;**166**:52-53. DOI: 10.1016/j.wneu.2022.07.059

[17] Katz JN, Zimmerman ZE, Mass H, Makhni MC. Diagnosis and management of lumbar spinal stenosis: A review. Journal of the American Medical Association. 2022;**327**(17):1688-1699. DOI: 10.1001/jama.2022.5921

[18] Barbero M, Schneebeli A, Koetsier E, Maino P. Myofascial pain syndrome and trigger points: Evaluation and treatment in patients with musculoskeletal pain. Current Opinion in Supportive and Palliative Care. 2019;**13**(3):270-276. DOI: 10.1097/SPC.0000000000000445

[19] Ceballos Laita L, Tejedor Cubillo C, Mingo Gómez T, Jiménez Del Barrio S. Effects of corrective, therapeutic exercise techniques on adolescent idiopathic scoliosis. A systematic review. Efectos de las técnicas de ejercicio terapéutico correctivo en la escoliosis idiopática del adolescente. Revisión sistemática. Archivos Argentinos de Pediatría. 2018;**116**(4):e582-e589. DOI: 10.5546/aap.2018.eng.e582

[20] Siracusa R, Paola RD, Cuzzocrea S, Impellizzeri D. Fibromyalgia: Pathogenesis, mechanisms, diagnosis and treatment options update. International Journal of Molecular Science. 2021;**22**(8):3891. DOI: 10.3390/ijms22083891

[21] Whale K, Gooberman-Hill R. The importance of sleep for people with chronic pain: Current insights and evidence. JBMR Plus. 2022;**6**(7):e10658. DOI: 10.1002/jbm4.10658

[22] Corp N, Mansell G, Stynes S, Wynne-Jones G, Morsø L, Hill JC, et al. Evidence-based treatment recommendations for neck and low back pain across Europe: A systematic review of guidelines. European Journal of Pain. 2021;**25**(2):275-295. DOI: 10.1002/ejp.1679

[23] Qaseem A, Wilt TJ, McLean RM, et al. Noninvasive treatments for acute, subacute, and chronic low Back pain: A Clinical Practice Guideline from the American College of Physicians. Annals of Internal Medicine. 2017;**166**(7):514-530. DOI: 10.7326/M16-2367

[24] Lang JK, Paykel MS, Haines KJ, Hodgson CL. Clinical practice guidelines for early mobilization in the ICU: A systematic review. Critical Care Medicine. 2020;**48**(11):e1121-e1128. DOI: 10.1097/CCM.0000000000004574

[25] Zhang L, Hu W, Cai Z, Liu J, Wu J, Deng Y, et al. Early mobilization of critically ill patients in the intensive care unit: A systematic review and meta-analysis. PLoS One. 2019;**14**(10):e0223185. DOI: 10.1371/journal.pone.0223185

[26] Simpson E, Hock E, Stevenson M, Wong R, Dracup N, Wailoo A, et al. What is the added value of ultrasound joint examination for monitoring synovitis in rheumatoid arthritis and can it be used to guide treatment decisions? A systematic review and cost-effectiveness analysis. Health Technology Assessment. 2018;**22**(20):1-258. DOI: 10.3310/hta22200

[27] Siegel P, Tencza M, Apodaca B, Poole JL. Effectiveness of occupational therapy interventions for adults with rheumatoid arthritis: A systematic review. American Journal of Occupational Therapy. 2017;**71**(1):7101180052p1-7101180050p11. DOI: 10.5014/ajot.2017.023176

[28] Hammond A, Meesters J, Niedermann K, Tennant A, Vliet Vlieland T, Tyson S, et al. Cross-cultural adaptation and psychometric testing of the Dutch and German versions of the Evaluation of Daily Activity Questionnaire in people with rheumatoid arthritis. Rheumatology International. 2021;**41**(5):951-964. DOI: 10.1007/s00296-020-04657-7

[29] Web. 1. Available from: https://www.google.ps/url?sa=i&url=https%3A%2F%2Fwww.amazon.com%2FTANDCF-Adjustable-Immobilizer-Arthritis-Osteoarthritis%2Fdp%2FB0863CX9CK&psig=AOvVaw3apaOauMgDIWcFNn8dQkHP&ust=1673204510213000&source=images&cd=vfe&ved=0CBAQjRxqFwoTCJCE0dSStvwCFQAAAAAdAAAAABAE

[30] Gavin JP, Rossiter L, Fenerty V, Leese J, Hammond A, Davidson E, et al. The role of occupational therapy for the self-management of rheumatoid arthritis: A protocol for a mixed methods systematic review. Musculoskeletal Care. 2022;**2022**:1665. DOI: 10.1002/msc.1665

[31] Rodziewicz TL, Houseman B, Hipskind JE. Medical Error Reduction and Prevention. Treasure Island (FL): StatPearls; 2022

[32] Web 2. Available from: https://m.media-amazon.com/images/W/WEBP_402378-T2/images/I/615vTun4u5L._SL1327_.jpg

[33] Fatoye F, Wright JM, Yeowell G, Gebrye T. Clinical and cost-effectiveness of physiotherapy interventions following total hip replacement: A systematic review and meta-analysis. Rheumatology International. 2020;**40**(9):1385-1398. DOI: 10.1007/s00296-020-04597-2

[34] Nakagawa S, Nakaishi M, Hashimoto M, Ito H, Yamamoto W, Nakashima R, et al. Effect of medication adherence on disease activity among Japanese patients with rheumatoid arthritis. PLoS One. 2018;**13**(11):e0206943. DOI: 10.1371/journal.pone.0206943

[35] Wollenhaupt J, Lee EB, Curtis JR, Silverfield J, Terry K, Soma K, et al. Safety and efficacy of tofacitinib for up to 9.5 years in the treatment of rheumatoid arthritis: Final results of a global, open-label, long-term extension study. Arthritis Research Therapy. 2019;**21**(1):89. DOI: 10.1186/s13075-019-1866-2

[36] García-Morales JM, Lozada-Mellado M, Hinojosa-Azaola A, Llorente L, Ogata-Medel M, Pineda-Juárez JA, et al. Effect of a dynamic exercise program in combination with Mediterranean diet on quality of life in women with rheumatoid arthritis. Journal of Clinical Rheumatology. 2020;**26**(75):S116-S122. DOI: 10.1097/RHU.0000000000001064

[37] Williams MA, Srikesavan C, Heine PJ, Bruce J, Brosseau L, Hoxey-Thomas N, et al. Exercise for rheumatoid arthritis of the hand. Cochrane Database System Review. 2018;7(7):CD003832. DOI: 10.1002/14651858.CD003832.pub3

[38] Web 3. Available from: https://www.google.ps/url?sa=i&url=https%3A%2F%2Fwww.researchgate.net%2Ffigure%2FExercises-for-strengthening-and-stretching_fig1_326660726&psig=AOvVaw3zEe0wfU5oY0djE0hStxVw&ust=1673205000516000&source=images&cd=vfe&ved=0CBAQjRxqFwoTCJCwor2UtvwCFQAAAAAdAAAAABAE

[39] García-Morales JM, Lozada-Mellado M, Hinojosa-Azaola A, Llorente L, Ogata-Medel M, Pineda-Juárez JA, et al. Effect of a dynamic

exercise program in combination with Mediterranean diet on quality of life in women with rheumatoid arthritis. Journal of Clinical Rheumatology. 2020;**26**(2):S116-S122. DOI: 10.1097/RHU.0000000000001064

[40] Web 4. Available from: http://tado.co.uk/wp-content/uploads/2014/05/rg1.jpg

[41] Peter WF, Swart NM, Meerhoff GA, Vliet Vlieland TPM. Clinical practice guideline for physical therapist management of people with rheumatoid arthritis. Physical Therapy. 2021;**101**(8): pzab127. DOI: 10.1093/ptj/pzab127

[42] Web 5. Available from: https://www.google.com/url?sa=i&url=https%3A%2F%2Fwww.phoenixrehabgroup.com%2Fparaffin-wax-bath-hand-physiotherapy.html&psig=AOvVaw0fomILsTHORGjBEktlhQgU&ust=1673205483747000&source=images&cd=vfe&ved=0CBAQjRxqFwoTCNi21KOWtvwCFQAAAAAdAAAAABAE

[43] Romero-Morales C, Bravo-Aguilar M, Abuín-Porras V, Almazán-Polo J, Calvo-Lobo C, Martínez-Jiménez EM, et al. Current advances and novel research on minimal invasive techniques for musculoskeletal disorders. Disease-a-Month. 2021 Oct;**67**(10):101210. DOI: 10.1016/j.disamonth.2021.101210

[44] Web 6. Available from: https://www.google.com/url?sa=i&url=https%3A%2F%2Fsolutionsphysicaltherapy.com%2Fphysical-therapy-treatments%2Felectrical-stimulation%2F&psig=AOvVaw15kimxwAQTvESyUoYGTmRY&ust=1673205533367000&source=images&cd=vfe&ved=0CBAQjRxqFwoTCNC7p7uWtvwCFQAAAAAdAAAAABAE

[45] Guo Q, Lin XM, Di Z, Zhang QA, Jiang S. Electroacupuncture ameliorates CUMS-induced depression-like behavior: Involvement of the glutamatergic system and apoptosis in rats. Combinatorial Chemistry & High Throughput Screening. 2021;**24**(7):996-1004. DOI: 10.2174/1386207323666201027121423

[46] Stausholm MB, Naterstad IF, Joensen J, Lopes-Martins RÁB, Sæbø H, Lund H, et al. Efficacy of low-level laser therapy on pain and disability in knee osteoarthritis: Systematic review and meta-analysis of randomised placebo-controlled trials. BMJ Open. 2019;**9**(10):e031142. DOI: 10.1136/bmjopen-2019-031142

[47] Web 7. Available from: https://www.google.com/url?sa=i&url=http%3A%2F%2Ffitptot.com%2Flaser-therapy%2F&psig=AOvVaw1SubwGhzff_tR2xU7d0ITr&ust=1673205587512000&source=images&cd=vfe&ved=0CBAQjRxqFwoTCMizotWWtvwCFQAAAAAdAAAAABAE

[48] Web 8. Available from: https://www.google.com/url?sa=i&url=https%3A%2F%2Fwww.forbes.com%2Fhealth%2Fbody%2Facupuncture-vs-acupressure%2F&psig=AOvVaw1B-brX-jJAZ68lfZ_AVQ0T&ust=1673205665562000&source=images&cd=vfe&ved=0CBAQjRxqFwoTCJi9svqWtvwCFQAAAAAdAAAAABAE

[49] Burmester GR, Álvaro-Gracia JM, Betteridge N, Calvo Alén J, Combe B, Durez P, et al. Evolving the comprehensive management of rheumatoid arthritis: Identification of unmet needs and development of practical and educational tools. Clinical and Experimental Rheumatology. 2020;**38**(6):1056-1067

[50] Lahiri M, Cheung PPM, Dhanasekaran P, Wong SR, Yap A,

Tan DSH, et al. Evaluation of a multidisciplinary care model to improve quality of life in rheumatoid arthritis: A randomised controlled trial. Quality of Life Research. 2022 Jun;**31**(6):1749-1759. DOI: 10.1007/s11136-021-03029-3

[51] Schulz M, Krohne B, Röder W, Sander K. Randomized, prospective, monocentric study to compare the outcome of continuous passive motion and controlled active motion after total knee arthroplasty. Technology and Health Care. 2018;**26**(3):499-506. DOI: 10.3233/THC-170850

[52] Bellew JW, Nolan T. Michlovitz's Modalities for Therapeutic Intervention. F. A. Davis Company; 2022

[53] Gunay Ucurum S, Kaya DO, Kayali Y, Askin A, Tekindal MA. Comparison of different electrotherapy methods and exercise therapy in shoulder impingement syndrome: A prospective randomized controlled trial. Acta Orthopaedica et Traumatologica Turcica. 2018;**52**(4):249-255. DOI: 10.1016/j.aott.2018.03.005

[54] Dantas LO, Salvini TF, McAlindon TE. Knee osteoarthritis: Key treatments and implications for physical therapy. Brazilian Journal of Physical Therapy. 2021;**25**(2):135-146. DOI: 10.1016/j.bjpt.2020.08.004

[55] Pieters L, Voogt L, Bury J, Littlewood C, Feijen S, Cavaggion C, et al. Rotator CUFF disorders: A survey of current physiotherapy practice in Belgium and the Netherlands. Musculoskeletal Science & Practice. 2019;**43**:45-51. DOI: 10.1016/j.msksp.2019.06.001

[56] Page P. Making the case for modalities: The need for critical thinking in practice. International Journal of Sports Physical Therapy. 2021;**16**(5):28326. DOI: 10.26603/001c.28326

[57] Page P, Mistretta C, Thompson J, Brittain K. Musculoskeletal Clinical Practice Guidelines Recommended Therapeutic Interventions. Baton Rouge, LA: American Physical Therapy Association -Louisiana; 2021

[58] Zadro J, O'Keeffe M, Maher C. Do physical therapists follow evidence-based guidelines when managing musculoskeletal conditions? Systematic review. BMJ Open. 2019;**9**(10):e032329. DOI: 10.1136/bmjopen-2019-032329

[59] Hsu JR, Mir H, Wally MK, Seymour RB, Orthopaedic Trauma Association Musculoskeletal Pain Task Force. Clinical practice guidelines for pain management in acute musculoskeletal injury. Journal of Orthopedic Trauma. 2019;**33**(5):e158-e182. DOI: 10.1097/BOT.0000000000001430

[60] Ellingsen DM, Napadow V, Protsenko E, Mawla I, Kowalski MH, Swensen D, et al. Brain mechanisms of anticipated painful movements and their modulation by manual therapy in chronic low back pain. Journal of Pain. 2018;**19**(11):1352-1365. DOI: 10.1016/j.jpain.2018.05.012

[61] Web 9. Available from: https://www.google.com/url?sa=i&url=https%3A%2F%2Fmusculoskeletalkey.com%2Fconcepts-of-joint-mobilization%2F&psig=AOvVaw1TW2thloMjNv8TvDdUOJMB&ust=1673205733585000&source=images&cd=vfe&ved=0CBAQjRxqFwoTCOjimJyXtvwCFQAAAAAdAAAAABAD

[62] Web 10. Available from: https://www.google.com/url?sa=i&url=https%3A%2F%2Faneskey.com%2Fmckenzie-method%2F&psig=AOvVaw1Na6kHFyY

RwnphwzETBRJI&ust=16732058022830 00&source=images&cd=vfe&ved=0CBA QjRxqFwoTCNC_8LuXtvwCFQAAAAA dAAAAABAE

[63] The Canadian Physio Student Manual Therapy in Physiotherapy Practice with Jesse Awenus. 2019. Available from: https://www.youtube.com/watch?v=g36vqjx5N-Q&app=desktop [Accessed: September 21, 2019]

[64] Web 11. Available from: https://www.google.com/url?sa=i&url=https%3A%2F%2Fmulliganproducts.eu%2Fabout-mulligan%2F&psig=AOvVaw0425PLYD1XUos5LN0vasVV&ust=1673205872559000&source=images&cd=vfe&ved=0CBAQjRxqFwoTCOiKlt6XtvwCFQAAAAAdAAAAABAJ

[65] Wellsandt E, Golightly Y. Exercise in the management of knee and hip osteoarthritis. Current Opinion in Rheumatology. 2018;**30**(2):151-159. DOI: 10.1097/BOR.0000000000000478

[66] Zeng CY, Zhang ZR, Tang ZM, Hua FZ. Benefits and mechanisms of exercise training for knee osteoarthritis. Frontiers in Physiology. 2021;**12**:794062. DOI: 10.3389/fphys.2021.794062

[67] Alcalde GE, Fonseca AC, Bôscoa TF, Gonçalves MR, Bernardo GC, Pianna B, et al. Effect of aquatic physical therapy on pain perception, functional capacity and quality of life in older people with knee osteoarthritis: Study protocol for a randomized controlled trial. Trials. 2017;**18**(1):317. DOI: 10.1186/s13063-017-2061-x

[68] Wang J, Chen X, Wang L, Zhang C, Ma J, Zhao Q. Does aquatic physical therapy affect the rehabilitation of breast cancer in women? A systematic review and meta-analysis of randomized controlled trials. PLoS One. 2022;**17**(8):e0272337. DOI: 10.1371/journal.pone.0272337

[69] Azeez M, Clancy C, O'Dwyer T, Lahiff C, Wilson F, Cunnane G. Benefits of exercise in patients with rheumatoid arthritis: A randomized controlled trial of a patient-specific exercise programme. Clinical Rheumatology. 2020;**39**(6):1783-1792. DOI: 10.1007/s10067-020-04937-4

[70] Lakomek HJ, Rudwaleit M, Hentschel A, Broge B, Abrolat J, Bessler F, et al. Qualität in der akutstationären Rheumatologic 2021 : Aktuelle Aspekte zum KOBRA-Qualitätslabel des Verbandes Rheumatologischer Akutkliniken (VRA e.V.) [Quality in acute inpatient rheumatology 2021 : Current aspects of the KOBRA quality label of the Association of Rheumatological Acute Care Clinics]. Rheumatology. 2021;**80**(8):758-770. DOI: 10.1007/s00393-021-01015-1

[71] Angulo J, El Assar M, Álvarez-Bustos A, Rodríguez-Mañas L. Physical activity and exercise: Strategies to manage frailty. Redox Biology. 2020;**35**:101513. DOI: 10.1016/j.redox.2020.101513

[72] Stefano SD. The Resistance Training Revolution: The no-Cardio Way to Burn Fat and Age-Proof your Body - in Only 60 Minutes a Week. Hachette Go; 2022

[73] Web 12. Available from: https://www.google.com/imgres?imgurl=https%3A%2F%2Fi0.wp.com%2Fisowalking.com%2Fwp-content%2Fuploads%2F2020%2F10%2Fcontraction_isometric.jpg&imgrefurl=https%3A%2F%2Fisowalking.com%2Ffaq%2F&tbnid=-3JXIfkKhZHRyM&vet=12ahUKEwjNt6yDmLb8AhW3UaQEHXEbCiIQMygCegUIARDoAQ..i&docid=hBje4Krs5loXTM&w=558&h=340&q=Isotonic%20Exercise&ved=2ahUKEwjNt6yDmLb8AhW3UaQEHXEbCiIQMygCegUIARDoAQ

[74] Web 13. Available from: https://www.google.com/url?sa=i&url=https%3A%2F%2Fwww.iprsmediquipe.com%2Fproducts%2Fbiodex-isokinetic-system-4%2F&psig=AOvVaw2bFtvDpUNK9PlMI3yC0rYW&ust=1673206054890000&source=images&cd=vfe&ved=0CBAQjRxqFwoTCND2wLSYtvwCFQAAAAAdAAAAABAE

[75] Ciprandi D, Zago M, Bertozzi F, Sforza C, Galvani C. Influence of energy cost and physical fitness on the preferred walking speed and gait variability in elderly women. Journal of Electromyography and Kinesiology. 2018 Dec;**43**:1-6. DOI: 10.1016/j.jelekin.2018.07.006

[76] Bosse C. Power training vs strength training - what is the difference between strength training and power training?. 2021. Available from: https://christianbosse.com/power-training-vs-strength-training-what-is-the-difference/ [Accessed: November 1, 2022]

[77] Englund DA, Kirn DR, Koochek A, Zhu H, Travison TG, Reid KF, et al. Nutritional supplementation with physical activity improves muscle composition in mobility-limited older adults, the VIVE2 study: A randomized, double-blind, placebo-controlled trial. Journal of Gerontology A Biological Science Medical Science. 2017;**73**(1):95-101. DOI: 10.1093/gerona/glx141

[78] Policy statement: Description of physical therapy. World Physiotherapy. (n.d.). Available from: https://world.physio/policy/ps-descriptionPT [Accessed: November 1, 2022]

[79] Bittermann A, Gao S, Rezvani S, Li J, Sikes KJ, Sandy J, et al. Oral ibuprofen interferes with cellular healing responses in a murine model of achilles tendinopathy. Journal of Musculoskeletal Disorder Treatment. 2018;**4**(2):049. DOI: 10.23937/2572-3243.1510049

[80] National Guideline Centre (UK). Evidence review for exercise for chronic primary pain: Chronic pain (primary and secondary) in over 16s: Assessment of all chronic pain and management of chronic primary pain: Evidence review E. London: National Institute for Health and Care Excellence (NICE); 2021

Chapter 5

# Guidelines for Prenatal and Postpartum Resistance Training

*Aly Matejka*


## Abstract

Resistance training can be a safe form of both prenatal and postnatal exercise with appropriate exercise selection and modification, safety considerations, and understanding of pregnancy and postpartum recovery. Clinicians, coaches, trainers, and pregnant and postpartum women themselves, should be made aware of common conditions that can impact exercise such as diastasis recti, prolapse, gestational diabetes, preeclampsia and pelvic floor dysfunction such as urinary incontinence. Prenatal modifications will be introduced broken down into trimesters and postpartum conditions and recovery will be discussed. This chapter will also discuss the positive impact resistance training can have on pregnant and postpartum women when it is performed utilizing general safety guidelines and contraindications are observed and respected.


**Keywords:** pregnant, postpartum, diastasis recti, prolapse, resistance training

## 1. Introduction

Historically, pregnant and postpartum women have been discouraged and even advised against partaking in physical activity for fear of harming or terminating their pregnancy [1]. With an explosion of research in prenatal and postpartum exercise in the last decade, not only has the myth that physical activity causes miscarriage been disproven, evidence to support prenatal and postpartum exercise as a contributing factor to improved maternal and fetal health has emerged [1–6]. Adherence to guidelines for prenatal and postpartum exercise, including resistance training, can ensure safe and active pregnancies and restorative postpartum recoveries. Topics discussed in this chapter include benefits and recommendations for prenatal exercise, general medical conditions that impact prenatal physical activity, contraindications and modifications for prenatal and postpartum exercise, common postpartum conditions that impact exercise and guidelines for postpartum exercise.

## 2. Benefits of and recommendations for exercise during pregnancy

Prenatal exercise has a plethora of benefits for both pregnant women and the fetus(es) they carry. Exercise during pregnancy has been shown to increase the incidence of vaginal delivery as well as lower the incidence of cesarean delivery, excessive gestational weight gain, gestational diabetes, gestational hypertensive disorders, preterm birth, and lower birth weight [1–6]. Additionally, prenatal exercise has a positive impact on healthy growth and improved cognition and intelligence of the baby after birth [3].

The American College of Obstetrics and Gynecology (ACOG) recommends 30 minutes of physical activity 5 days a week for pregnant women [1, 6–9]. Pregnant women with uncomplicated pregnancies, or pregnancies free of medical conditions that are deemed unsafe by their obstetrician, are safe to engage in both resistance training and aerobic activities. Contraindications for prenatal exercise will be further discussed in Section 2.4. It is important to note that according to the CDC, only 15% of American women meet these recommendations for prenatal physical activity [1]. Identified barriers to prenatal exercise include lack of energy and becoming too uncomfortable especially in the third trimester in addition to lack of education in safe prenatal exercise practices [1, 10, 11]. Despite its safety, only 11% of pregnant women engage in resistance training during their pregnancy [4, 12]. Acute bouts of resistance exercise are consistently associated with increased feelings of energy and decreased feelings of fatigue in pregnant women during the second and third trimesters [11].

Historically, physical activity was deemed unsafe for pregnant women for fear that it would cause a miscarriage or have negative impact on the developing fetus [1, 6, 8]. This view could be largely attributed to the lack of understanding of the physiological maternal adaptations throughout the 40 weeks of pregnancy. Physiological maternal adaptations include 50% increase in plasma, 40% increase in red blood cell volume, 40% increase in cardiac output in the late second trimester that remains stable until delivery, 40–50% increase in renal blood flow starting at 6 weeks gestation, 35–50% increase in tidal volume, 5% increase and lung capacity, and 10–20% increase in oxygen consumption [8]. All of these adaptations demonstrate the ability of the pregnant body to accommodate the growing fetus while also maintaining physical activity.

## 2.1 Strenuous exercise during pregnancy

While physical activity is both safe and beneficial, there are consequences for strenuous activity (95–100% $Vo_2max$ to the point of exhaustion) [8]. Such strenuous activity may result in elevated maternal sympathetic response, reduced maternal placental blood flow, elevated maternal lactic acid, reduced glucose delivery, lowered maternal pH, increased uterine contractility, and reduced fetal oxygen [8]. Therefore, it is not recommended that pregnant women perform repeated bouts of extremely strenuous exercises at 95–100% of their $Vo_2max$ or continue long duration workouts at a high level of perceived effort [8].

Women who are considered "untrained" can safely exercise at a moderate intensity 70–75% of $Vo_2max$, while trained women can handle up to 85–90% of $Vo_2max$ [8].

## 2.2 Prenatal general medical conditions and their impact on physical activity

Two common prenatal medical conditions that can impact a pregnant woman's ability to continue safe exercise are gestational diabetes and preeclampsia [13–15]. These conditions can develop during pregnancy and should be carefully monitored by the pregnant woman's primary care physician or obstetrician.

Gestational diabetes is impaired glucose intolerance that is diagnosed for the first time during pregnancy and is associated with other prenatal conditions such as preeclampsia, hypertension, preterm birth and higher incidence of induced labor and cesarean delivery [13, 14]. It occurs in 2–10% of pregnancies and does not have any symptoms. Healthcare providers routinely test for gestational diabetes around 24–28 weeks gestation. If diagnosed, the pregnant woman will be advised to check her blood sugar, modify her diet, and partake in physical activity.

Moderate-intensity exercise training during pregnancy is associated with a lower incidence of gestational diabetes and reduced maternal weight gain [3, 6, 13, 14]. Prenatal physical activity yields the best results in managing gestational diabetes and maternal weight gain when performed in a combination aerobic and resistance training. Additionally, the benefits of physical activity are greater when started in the first trimester [6].

Preeclampsia is a serious high blood pressure condition that develops during pregnancy usually after 20 weeks gestation. It occurs in 3–7% of pregnancies and is more commonly seen in 1st time mothers, mothers who are black or of African descent, and those with a history of high blood pressure or thyroid conditions [15]. Preeclampsia can develop without symptoms and can change suddenly and drastically so it is important to regularly monitor maternal blood pressure throughout pregnancy. This condition should be closely monitored by the pregnant woman's healthcare provider and exercise may or may not be recommended depending on the severity of the condition. Blood pressure medication may be prescribed to lower pressure during pregnancy and preeclampsia usually resolves after birth.

### 2.3 Contraindications and warning signs to terminate prenatal exercise

ACOG outlines absolute contraindications to prenatal exercise that include; significant heart or lung disease, incompetent cervix, multiple gestations at risk for premature labour, persistent second or third trimester bleeding, placenta previa after twenty-six weeks, premature labour during this pregnancy, ruptured membranes, and pregnancy-induced hypertension [9]. All of these conditions pose significant risk to maternal and fetal health and therefore should be considered absolute contraindications for exercise unless otherwise determined by the pregnant woman's obstetrician (**Table 1**).

There are also environmental conditions that should be considered as they can have adverse impacts on prenatal exercise. Higher altitude creates challenges in

| Contraindications to prenatal exercise | Warning signs to stop prenatal exercise |
|---|---|
| • Significant heart or lung disease | • Shortness of breath before exercising |
| • Incompetent cervix | • Dizziness |
| • Multiple gestations at risk for premature labor | • Headache |
| • Persistent second or third trimester bleeding | • Chest pain |
| • Placenta previa after twenty-six weeks | • Calf pain or swelling |
| • Premature labor during this pregnancy | • Vaginal bleeding |
| • Ruptured membranes | • Preterm labor |
| • Pregnancy-induced hypertension | • Decreased fetal movement |
| | • Amniotic fluid leakage |
| | • Muscle weakness |

**Table 1.**
*Contraindications to and warning signs to stop prenatal exercise [9].*

handling exercise load for the pregnant woman and warrants caution. It is recommended that pregnant women stay in a more moderate heart rate zone, 50–60% max heart rate, for a shorter duration- about 20 min [8, 9]. Prenatal exercise in high temperatures can have adverse effects on maternal and fetal health. Because increased fetal heart rate correlates with higher maternal body temperatures, maternal body temperature, especially with strenuous exercise, should be closely monitored. Prolonged exercise of more than 45 min can result in elevated core maternal and fetal temperature and increased uterine contractions, leading to preterm labor [8].

While physical activity is safe for most pregnancies, there are definitive warning signs to terminate or cease prenatal exercise. Some warning signs are those that are applied to any person working out such as shortness of breath before exercising, dizziness, headache, chest pain, calf pain or swelling. Others are very specific to pregnancy; vaginal bleeding, preterm labor, decreased fetal movement, amniotic fluid leakage, muscle weakness. All of these symptoms should be treated as indicators that exercise should be stopped immediately and reported to the pregnant woman's obstetrician [9].

## 3. Exercise modification for pregnant women

The 40 weeks of pregnancy are commonly broken down into three trimesters that serve as mile markers for both fetal development and maternal changes. In regards to prenatal exercise, the trimesters serve as general time frames for when modifications need to be made for safe exercise practice.

### 3.1 The first trimester

In general, women experiencing healthy, uncomplicated pregnancies do not require much exercise modification in the first trimester. For most women, the first trimester is marked by mild to extreme fatigue [11]. Scaling back on exercise volume to reduce fatigue can be a useful strategy until energy levels return in the second trimester. Nausea is also very common in the first trimester making maintenance of adequate nutrition and physical activity difficult.

### 3.2 The second trimester

Upon entering the second trimester, more exercise modifications are necessary to accommodate the expanding uterus and pregnant belly. Modifications are also necessary to help manage the development of diastasis recti and bearing down into the pelvic floor which can ultimately lead to pelvic organ prolapse.

Diastasis recti, or abdominal separation, is a normal and necessary adaptation for the pregnant body. As the uterus expands and the fetus grows, the two rectus abdominal muscles will separate to create more space. Diastasis recti also involves the thinning and stretching of the linea alba, or the connective tissue between the two rectus abdominal muscles [16, 17]. It is measured by both the width between the two separated rectus abdominis muscles and the degree of tissue thinning of the linea alba. Diastasis recti is prevalent in 33% of pregnant women at 21 weeks gestation and 100% of pregnant women at 35 weeks gestation [16]. While diastasis recti is necessary prenatal accommodation, it should be managed appropriately to limit the amount of separation and thinning.

Important considerations in limiting diastasis recti during pregnancy include posture, body awareness, and intra abdominal pressure management. Pregnant women should be coached on being more mindful of how they are carrying themselves and maintaining posture throughout the day. Pregnancy tends to invoke an anterior pelvic tilt, therefore placing additional stress on the anterior core and the separating rectus abdominis muscles and thinning linea alba [18]. Placing unnecessary pressure on these structures when getting up from the seated position or utilizing a "crunch" to sit up can also exacerbate diastasis recti.

Specific modifications that need to be made starting in the second trimester to help manage diastasis recti include removing front loading exercises from the pregnant woman's workout routine. Front loading exercises include crunches, planks, pull-ups, push-ups, and leg lifts. Front loading exercises generate excessive intra abdominal pressure that presses on the linea alba and rectus abdominis muscles causing a more significant diastasis recti [19].

Pelvic organ prolapse, or more commonly referred to simply as prolapse, occurs when pelvic floor muscles and ligaments stretch and weaken and no longer provide enough support for the uterus. As a result, the uterus slips down into or protrudes out of the vagina [20]. The pelvic floor muscles and connective tissues are responsible for supporting pelvic organs such as the bowels and bladder and uterus and vagina in females. Additionally they provide the contractor mechanism for the anal canal, urethra, and vagina.

As a pregnancy progresses, the uterus expands and becomes heavier placing increased strain on the pelvic floor. If the pregnant woman exerts additional downward pressure into the pelvic floor such as excessive pushing to have a bowel movement or bracing and bearing down with lifting a heavy object, the pelvic floor tissue may not be able to withstand the pressure and prolapse can result. Prolapse can be avoided during pregnancy by properly managing intra abdominal pressure when lifting, removing front loading exercises from the workout routine, and consulting a healthcare provider if persistent constipation occurs during the pregnancy.

Another modification to consider upon entering the second trimester is performing exercises in the supine position. Extended time spent in the supine position can cause venous obstruction in some pregnant women [21–23]. The weight of the uterus and fetus can compress both the superior vena cava and the aorta while in the supine position. This can reduce blood flow to the uterus and make the pregnant woman feel dizzy, light headed, and possibly nauseous. Therefore it is recommended that pregnant women do not lie flat on their back after the first trimester but rather utilize an inclined position in lieu of the full supine position. Some modifications that can be made for exercises commonly performed in the supine position include; seated deadbugs, incline chest press, and being creative with the kneeling or half kneeling positions for different shoulder fly movements.

### 3.3 The third trimester

Further modifications are needed throughout the third trimester as the uterus expands, the fetus grows larger and heavier, abdominal separation increases, the pelvic floor undergoes more stress, hormones change to relax ligaments to prepare for delivery, movement becomes more challenging for the pregnant woman, and fatigue increases.

If the pregnant woman has been running throughout her pregnancy, she is welcome to continue to do so but it may be beneficial to phase out running as the stress it imposes on the pelvic floor may become more problematic as her due date approaches.

Urinary incontinence, or the involuntary leaking of urine, becomes more likely in the third trimester. An estimated 37% of women experience urinary incontinence during pregnancy and it is most common in the third trimester [24]. Running and jumping will increase the incidence of urinary incontinence during pregnancy as it significantly increases the stress on the pelvic floor [2] which is already undergoing increased stress from the weight of the uterus and growing fetus. Other lower-impact modes of cardiovascular training should be considered to replace running such as walking, swimming, stairmaster, elliptical, upper body ergometer, etc.

There are six key pregnancy hormones that help regulate the female body to maintain a normal pregnancy. The six key hormones are human chorionic gonadotropin (hCG), progesterone, estrogen, prolactin, oxytocin, and relaxin. For the purposes of this chapter we will focus only on relaxin and its role during pregnancy as it has the most direct impact on exercise and resistance training.

Relaxin, a peptide hormone of the insulin-like growth factor family, has been associated with collagen remodeling. It is secreted by the corpus luteum in the ovary and by the placenta beginning around the 10th–12th week of pregnancy [25]. In addition to inhibiting uterine contractions to prevent preterm birth, relaxing blood vessels, increasing blood flow to the placenta and kidneys, and softening and lengthening the cervix during birth, relaxin relaxes the joints of the pelvis in preparation for delivery [25, 26]. It is believed that relaxin increases pelvic laxity, and predisposes separation of the pubic symphysis, by altering the structure of collagen [25].

Pelvic and sacroiliac joint (SIJ) pain are common complaints of pregnant women particularly in their third trimester and may be attributed to the changes in the pelvic region due to increased relaxin levels [25, 27, 28]. This will lead to a need for exercise modification to reduce pelvic and SIJ pain. Modification suggestions include decreasing or eliminating single leg exercises such as single leg deadlifts and decreasing exercises performed with wide legs such as plie squats. It is also recommended to increase glute and hamstring strength to help stabilize the pelvis.

Lastly, for women still engaging in resistance training in the third trimester are encouraged to continue pending that they feel comfortable and motivated to do so. Scaling back is also appropriate as the pregnant woman will be experiencing greater challenges with movement, discomfort, and lack of energy. General guidelines to help maintain resistance training include decreasing barbell lifts especially if she is experiencing difficulties navigating her large belly and maintaining balance, and utilizing free weights and bands as necessary.

### 3.4 Guidelines for prenatal resistance training

Resistance training is a safe mode of physical exercise for women experiencing uncomplicated pregnancies and have been cleared by their healthcare provider to do so [12–14, 29]. It can be beneficial in maintaining current strength, posture, and mood during pregnancy. When done properly, without creating excessive intra abdominal pressure or bearing down into the pelvic floor, it can prepare the body for labor and help maintain pelvic stability.

When designing a prenatal resistance training program, it is important to consider that not only does each woman experience pregnancy differently, it can also vary widely with each pregnancy in the same woman. This makes it exceedingly difficult to create an all-encompassing prenatal resistance training plan that is appropriate and realistic for all women and all pregnancies. Some women will be able to continue resistance training at a high level for their entire pregnancy. Some will feel the need to scale back almost immediately. While it varies widely, there are some concepts and components that can be applied to all prenatal resistance training.

Front loading exercise, as previously mentioned, should be removed from physical activity and lifting routines by the start of the second trimester. This will help decrease unnecessary pressure on the linea alba and pelvic floor to manage diastasis recti and prevent pelvic floor dysfunction and prolapse during pregnancy.

Equipment selection will also be an important consideration as pregnancy progresses. As the pregnant belly continues to grow, lifting a barbell may not be comfortable or safe- ensuring that there is adequate clearance from the belly while lifting and lowering the barbell will need to be a top priority to prevent dropping the bar on the pregnant belly [2]. Balance will also be altered as the pelvis tilts anteriorly and the pregnant belly expands 18]. It may not be advisable for some pregnant women experiencing balance changing to lift the barbell even if she is an experienced lifter. Proper monitoring of balance changes should be completed periodically to determine if specific equipment selections are safe. Dumbbells and resistance bands are safe alternatives to heavier equipment if balance issues are present [2].

The intensity of prenatal exercise will vary from woman to woman depending on her level of physical fitness before becoming pregnant and the goals she has in maintaining that fitness. The American College of Sports Medicine (ASCM) defines moderate exercise as d as exercise of 3–4 METS or any activity that is equivalent in difficulty to brisk walking without any reason to alter the recommendation for pregnant women [30]. It should be noted that the allowance for intensity for pregnant women wishing to maintain or progress physical fitness throughout pregnancy is increased without cause for safety concerns in uncomplicated pregnancies. The ACSM recommends that intensity should be 60–90% of maximal heart rate or 50–85% of either maximal oxygen uptake or heart rate reserve. The lower end of these ranges (60–70% of maximal heart rate or 50–60% of maximal oxygen uptake) appears to be appropriate for most pregnant women who did not engage in regular exercise before pregnancy, and the upper part of these ranges should be considered for those who wish to continue to maintain fitness during pregnancy [30].

ACOG recommends the use of ratings of perceived exertion (RPE) in addition to heart rate suggesting the use of Borg's conventional 6–20-point scale, with 12–14 (a rating of 13 corresponds to a subjective rating of "somewhat hard") identified as the RPE range to apply in pregnancy [30, 31]. Occasional higher intensity cardiovascular activities may be completed for short time periods, but time spent exceeding the RPE ranges of 5–7 should be limited as the increased pressure directly impacts the health of the pelvic floor [2]. Historically there was a prenatal maximum heart rate limit of 140 bpm that has since been discredited by ACOG. Observing this unsupported heart rate maximum is not necessary [32].

While no universal prenatal resistance training protocol currently exists due to the wide variability in previous lifting experience, pre-pregnancy physical fitness levels, and prenatal medical conditions, The ACSM does provide basic guidelines for safety measures. In general, the ACSM does not recommend using a one repetition maximum (1-RM) with pregnant women [31]. It is suggested that clinicians, coaches, and trainers use the Oddvar Holten diagram to make a 1-RM prediction to guide resistance training. For example, the clinician, coach or trainer, makes an estimation of the weight that can be lifted for 10–20 times; the number of repetitions that can be maximally performed is registered; the percentage of intensity can than be looked up in the Oddvar Holten diagram, seen in **Figure 1**, at the number of repetitions and 1RM can be computed by the formula as seen in **Figure 2** [31].

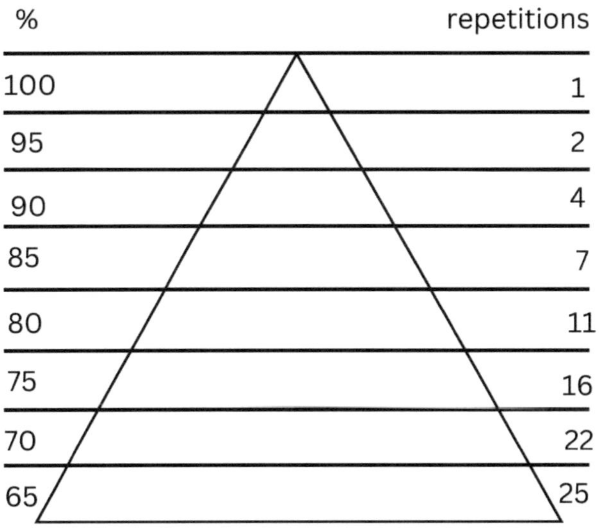


**Figure 1.**
*Oddvar Holten diagram.*

$$\frac{A\text{ kg} \times 100\%}{B\ \%} = 1\text{ R.M.}$$

**Figure 2.**
*Formula. A: lifted weight; B: percentage of intensity.*

The most important consideration for prenatal resistance training is determining if the pregnant woman is properly managing intra abdominal pressure and is not bearing down into the pelvic floor. Pregnant women who engage in prenatal resistance training should be educated on how to manage intra abdominal pressure by utilizing proper breathing and bracing technique rather than a breath-holding technique. Pregnant women should breathe through their lift without holding their breath or simulating a valsalva maneuver as it generates significant pressure in the abdomen [33]. This pressure also can go directly down into the pelvic floor leading to dysfunction or prolapse. It is estimated that 46% of women had some degree of prolapse at 36 week gestation [34], making it a common concern especially if continuing resistance training throughout pregnancy.

Generally, resistance training movement selections should be made with the intention of focusing on the outlined goals of the pregnant woman and with respect to her energy levels, nausea, and other common pregnancy symptoms. If the goal is to maintain a moderate level of physical activity during pregnancy, the focus of resistance training should be on postural endurance and endurance with full body movements. Resistance training should take place at least 2 days in a week with a selection of movements desired by the patient and clinician, coach, or trainer [2]. Movements that focus on pelvic stabilization such as squats and lunges, postural strength and endurance such as rows and flys, and work in the quadruped position such as bird dogs are all encouraged to be utilized in prenatal resistance training [2].

## 4. Postpartum recovery and common postpartum conditions

Before discussing postpartum exercise, it is important to have a solid understanding of the postpartum recovery process and common postpartum conditions that impact a woman's return to exercise. No two postpartum experiences are alike and there are a plethora of different conditions that may or may not occur after every delivery. All of the following conditions should be carefully considered by the clinician, coach, or trainer and discussed thoroughly with the postpartum woman and her medical provider if necessary, before designing a postpartum exercise program.

Although commonly thought of as the space between the vagina and the anus, the female perineum is a diamond shaped structure spanning from the pubic symphysis and the coccyx. The perineum is essential for supporting the pelvic floor and when tearing occurs in childbirth, damage can be done to muscle, fascia, veins, arteries, and nerves housed in the perineum. Tears range in severity from a 1st degree tear (first layer of skin around the vagina) to 4th degree tear (extends from the vagina to the anus). A 2nd degree tear is most common and 85% of women experience some degree of tearing in a vaginal delivery [35]. Tearing can impact the perineum's ability to support the pelvic floor and unresolved trauma can lead to urinary and fecal incontinence and prolapse [36]. This type of birth injury can have a direct impact on postpartum physical activity and should be a consideration for program design.

C-sections are performed when vaginal delivery is too risky for the pregnant woman or the fetus, when labor has become complicated or fails to progress, or can be elected through consultation with the patient and obstetrician. This surgery involves cutting through skin, fat, fascia, and the uterus. Abdominal muscles are separated, not cut.Incisions are generally 12–17 cm, or 4.5–6.5 inches and the resulting scar tissue can make the surrounding skin and fascia tight and restricted [37]. The scar can also be painful, tender, sensitive, or lacking in sensation. This will have an impact on the recovery and return to physical activity timeline. As a general rule, no physical activity should occur before the incision has closed and clearance from a healthcare provider has been obtained.

Arguably, the condition most commonly exacerbated by premature return to postpartum physical activity is prolapse. At six weeks postpartum, 83% of women have some degree of prolapse and at 7–11 weeks postpartum, 52% of women develop a new prolapse, or a prolapse that was not present at the 6 week checkup [38]. Resistance training and running can generate intra abdominal pressure that pushes directly down on the pelvic floor that creates or exacerbates prolapse [2]. Prolapse can be avoided by gradually progressing the training program and scaling back when symptoms dictate. Prolapse and its impact on physical activity is related to perineum tearing and resulting scar tissue, pelvic floor resting tone (how tight or loose the pelvic floor muscles are), and whether or not the woman experienced prolapse or pelvic floor dysfunction during pregnancy. All of these factors should be considered before returning to physical activity.

Postpartum women commonly experience urinary (and sometimes fecal) incontinence with physical activity [2, 39]. It is referred to as stress urinary incontinence and is the leaking of urine without an urge and is brought on by a stressor such as running or jumping. When the muscles of the pelvic floor are not strong enough to support the bladder and/or contract the muscles that tighten the opening of the urethra, urine may leak when a stressor is introduced. It is important to recognize that while urinary incontinence is common in postpartum women, it is not normal. It is a sign of pelvic floor dysfunction and needs to be rehabilitated as any other injury before physical activity begins or continues. Urinary leakage needs to be acknowledged as a symptom of dysfunction and a potential precursor to prolapse and a sign that running and resistance training may not be appropriate until proper pelvic floor rehabilitation has taken place [2]. Pelvic floor therapy is not recommended to pregnant or postpartum women as a standard of care in the United States, leaving women to self advocate for such treatment [2]. Informed clinicians, coaches, and trainers could be instrumental in recognizing these signs of pelvic floor dysfunction and recommending or referring a client or patient for pelvic floor therapy.

Diastasis recti, while a normal adaptation of pregnancy, needs to be rehabilitated and permitted to heal before strenuous physical activity occurs. Some natural healing of the linea alba and surrounding fascia does occur spontaneously in the early postpartum weeks [17]. An estimated 60% of postpartum women have a diastasis at 6 weeks postpartum which decreases to 32% of women at 12 weeks postpartum [16]. There are several factors that impact the severity of diastasis recti including genetic factors related to collagen and elastin, advanced maternal age, ethnicity, number of pregnancies carried to term, pregnancies with multiple fetuses, high birth weight, and maternal weight gain [8, 16, 19]. All of these factors can impact the amount of spontaneous healing that is possible in addition to postpartum hormonal changes that regulate tissue healing.

Postpartum hormones are responsible for maternal recovery but also prepare the woman's body to produce breast milk. The four key postpartum hormones are estrogen, progesterone, oxytocin, and prolactin [40]. Relaxin is also a hormone produced in pregnancy that remains present in the postpartum body. For the purposes of this chapter, we will primarily focus on postpartum estrogen and relaxin levels as they have the greatest impact on physical activity.

Estrogen level dramatically drops to 10% of the prenatal value and reaches its lowest value by 7 days postpartum [40]. If the postpartum woman breastfeeds the newborn, estrogen levels will remain low until ceasing breastfeeding. The American Academy of Pediatrics recommends exclusive breastfeeding for the first 6 months and urges greater support for mothers to nurse until at least 1 year of age [41], so this could be a significant period of low estrogen. This has a profound effect on postpartum tissue healing as estrogen is directly linked to tissue healing [42]. Low levels of estrogen may delay perineal tearing and c-section incisions. Additionally, long term suppressed estrogen due to breastfeeding may delay the soft tissue healing of the linea alba in regards to diastasis recti healing.

Relaxin, the hormone responsible for relaxing the ligaments in the pelvis in preparation for delivery, remains present for 12 months after delivery and longer if breastfeeding [43]. This means that women who do choose to breastfeed will have the effect of relaxin; ligament relaxation and laxity, possible SIJ pain, and pelvic pain. There is also some evidence to suggest that increased levels of relaxin in postpartum women can delay healing of diastasis recti because relaxin is designed to increase soft tissue laxity [17, 43]. The linea alba serves as the anchor for the rectus abdominis and transverse abdominis and if its tissue integrity is compromised by relaxin, abdominal strengthening and healing of the diastasis recti may be delayed [17].

After delivery, the hormone prolactin will prompt milk production. If a woman chooses to breastfeed, levels of prolactin will rise and fall in proportion to nipple stimulation [40]. When a postpartum woman's milk comes in, they can experience engorgement of the breasts which can range from uncomfortable to painful. Direct nursing or using a breast pump will relieve the engorgement. Breastfeeding continues on a supply and demand basis, meaning that the more the baby nurses (or the more milk that is pumped) the more the breasts will produce and if the baby nurses less (or less is pumped) then the supply will go down [41]. This process will fluctuate over the course of breastfeeding until weaning is initiated and eventually prolactin levels drop and milk ceases to be produced. For women who choose not to breastfeed or cannot breastfeed, prolactin levels usually return to normal around 7 days postpartum [40].

It is to be expected that new mothers will experience significant sleep loss and fatigue following the birth of their baby. Postpartum women experience disrupted sleep patterns that can lead to sleep disturbances and sleep deprivation. Common postpartum sleep patterns include lack of nocturnal sleep that is replaced by daytime sleep. Many women report that sleep disturbances continued well past the 3 month postpartum mark [44, 45]. Sleep disturbances and sleep deprivation are closely intertwined with depressive symptoms and postpartum depression. Postpartum depression is most common 3 weeks after delivery up until the 6 month mark but can present later as well [46, 47]. Women who experience miscarriage or stillbirth are at a higher risk of developing postpartum depression and those experiencing preterm delivery are at an increased risk for posttraumatic stress disorders [47].

### 4.1 The postpartum checkup

At six weeks postpartum, women are seen by their healthcare provider, usually the obstetrician's office that oversaw the pregnancy, labor and delivery. At this postpartum checkup the provider will check the incision if a c-section was performed and the perineum will be checked if tearing occurred or stitches were used. The uterus will also be externally evaluated and the breasts will be examined. The provider will also do a general medical assessment in taking blood pressure, height, weight, and heart rate. The postpartum patient will also complete a survey to assess for postpartum depression.

Barring any major red flags, the postpartum woman is medically cleared to resume physical activity, usually with very little guidance as to where to begin or how to progress safely. Many women incorrectly assume they are ready to return to running and resistance training at this point. There are several reasons why returning to physical activity after giving birth needs to be done as a gradual progression including; perineum tears, c-section incisions, healing prolapse, urinary and fecal incontinence, healing diastasis recti, hormonal changes, breastfeeding and changes to the breasts, fatigue, and mental health considerations.

### 4.2 Postpartum exercise readiness guidelines

The first step in returning to postpartum exercise is gaining clearance from the obstetrician or healthcare provider. Even after a postpartum woman is cleared by her physician, it is highly recommended that clinicians, coaches, and trainers utilize a physical activity readiness questionnaire (PAR-Q) to identify contraindications for postpartum exercise. These questionnaires are completed by the patient before any physical activity begins. If contraindications for exercise are identified, the patient should be referred back to her physician to address any health concerns [2]. If no contraindications are identified, the postpartum conditions outlined in the previous section should be carefully considered while creating an exercise routine (**Table 2**).

Contraindications and signs that exercise should stop for postnatal exercise include; postpartum bleeding (lochia) changes color, heavier flow, or starts again

- What type of delivery did you have, vaginal or c-section?
- Are you breastfeeding?
- Did you have your postnatal check-up?
- Did your healthcare provider clear you for physical activity at your postnatal checkup?
- Currently or during pregnancy, have you suffered any of the following?
    - Pubic symphysis dysfunction, sacroiliac joint dysfunction, or pelvic pain
    - Tearing/episiotomy or problem with stitches
    - Urinary or fecal incontinence
    - C-section wound discomfort
    - Diastasis recti (abdominal muscle separation)
    - Prolapse
    - Bleeding during or after exercise
    - Gestational diabetes

**Table 2.**
*Sample postpartum physical activity readiness questions [2].*

after stopping, feelings of heaviness or bulging in the vagina, leaking urine during or after exercise, pelvic pain, bulging or doming of the abdomen during exercise or discomfort afterwards [48], increased fatigue, dizziness or lightheadedness, difficulty breathing, chest pain, and pain or discomfort around the c-section scar or perineum stitches if applicable.

## 5. Foundational postpartum physical activity timeline

While prenatal exercise is largely scaling back as the pregnancy progresses, postpartum exercise is the reverse process; exercise needs to be gradually and progressively implemented over time. Every postpartum woman recovers differently and recovery is dependent upon several factors including her labor and delivery experience, health before and after delivery, mental health concerns, postpartum support, and the health and wellbeing of her new baby and other children and family members. Therefore, it is difficult to assign specific physical activity milestones to all postpartum women. However there are safety precautions and logical sequencing of rehabilitation and return to physical activity that can be utilized to ensure safe postpartum exercise.

For the purpose of this textbook, a focus on resistance training will take persistence over details about all types of physical activity including cardiovascular exercise. Historically, it has been advised that postpartum women do absolutely no exercise or mobility work in the first 6 weeks after delivery with many healthcare professionals still insisting on this outdated practice. Then they would be cleared for all activity at the 6 week postpartum check-up leaving a very wide gap in physical activity readiness leading to pain or injury of postpartum women returning to exercise. Updated protocols for postpartum physical activity do include foundational movements that can be performed in the early postpartum weeks to encourage healing and better prepare women for a return to physical activity [2].

In the very early postpartum weeks, weeks 0–2, if a woman wants to engage in movements, mobilization and postural movements need to be the primary focus.

Some examples can be encouraging anterior and posterior pelvic tilts for postural alignment and light standing open kinetic chain movements. In weeks 3–4 postpartum, women can initiate short duration (less than 15 min) walks as well movements such as transverse abdominis engagement and glute bridges. In weeks 5–6 postpartum, an increase in walking duration (less than 30 min) can be implemented as well as muscular activities such as standing and quadruped hip abduction and extension, double leg calf raises, as well as sit to stand movements [2]. The intensity of all movements during the first 6 weeks postpartum should be kept at an RPE of 0–2 [2].

Upon clearance at the 6 week postpartum checkup, postpartum women can progress to muscular strength tasks either with body weight or with additional weights if appropriate. These muscular strength tasks can include squats, single leg sit to stand, and single leg calf raises. It should be noted that most recent evidence suggests that impact exercises such as running and jumping should be postponed until weeks 8–10 postpartum. Before doing so, gradual dynamic movements should be progressed in the exercise routine and can include single leg calf raises, single leg hop down from a step, single leg hopping, and jumping in place [2]. It is recommended that RPE during tasks should be maintained under a 6 [2].

It is also highly recommended that every postpartum woman see a pelvic floor therapist at least once after delivery. After clearance from the healthcare provider at the 6 week checkup is an ideal time to seek pelvic floor therapy as they will be able to perform an internal examination. The pelvic floor therapist can determine if there are any contraindications to advancing further into exercise such as pelvic floor dysfunction or prolapse that could be made worse by more stressful physical activity [2].

Most recent evidence suggests that 13 weeks postpartum is a safe point to return to running and sport activity given that the postpartum woman has progressed throughout other stages of postpartum recovery and exercise without complication [2]. Resistance training can begin to safely progress into more sets, repetitions, or weight depending on the lifting experience of the postpartum woman and her recovery process thus far.

## 6. Guidelines for postpartum resistance training

Upon successful progression through foundational physical activity milestones, postpartum women are capable of returning to resistance training. It is recommended that clinicians, coaches, and trainers discuss specific goals and exercise expectations with their postpartum patients or clients so they design exercise plans that progress realistically in conjunction with their patient or clients needs and desires.

Recall that beginning in the second trimester, front loading exercises including crunches, planks, pull-ups, push-ups, and leg lifts, were removed from exercise routines. Progressive reintroduction of these movements can be accomplished safely if the postpartum woman is monitored and educated on abdominal doming or bulging, diastasis recti and intra abdominal pressure management.

Diastasis recti can be assessed very simply through self-examination by lying on the floor with knees bent and feet on the ground. Then, while performing a small crunch with head and shoulders off the ground, palpate the linea alba from distal sternum to the pubic bone noting tissue tension (or lack thereof) and also noting the distance between the two rectus abdominis muscles. When the distance between the two rectus abdominis muscles exceeds 2 finger widths there is considered to be a diastasis [19, 43]. Tissue tension is an important factor for determining severity of a diastasis as tissue integrity needs to be insured for proper biomechanical function. If a diastasis recti exists, front loading exercises in particular will need to be carefully prescribed and pressure management education will need to be administered. The clinician, coach, or trainer will need to watch for abdominal doming or bulging of the lower abdomen as it is an indicator that pressure is not being properly managed.

A common cause of abdominal doming or bulging in postpartum women is a lack of connection or firing of the transverse abdominis. These muscles are responsible for maintaining abdominal wall tension in order to stabilize the spine and the pelvis before movement of the limbs occurs [49]. Because the transverse abdominis muscles co-contract with the muscles of the pelvic floor [49, 50] and have altered firing patterns after pregnancy [49], it may take significant retraining to properly engage these muscles to restore a functioning core. Abdominal doming and bulging are an indicator that the transverse abdominis muscles may not be contracting or may not be contracting the proper sequence in relation to the rectus abdominis and oblique muscles [49]. Retraining the transverse abdominis is the first step in reintroducing front loading abdominal exercises to the postpartum woman.

Equipment selection and the amount of weight lifted are very important factors to consider when designing postpartum exercise plans. Equipment selection should follow a logical progression with a recommendation for starting with bodyweight exercises, followed by resistance band use, followed by hand weight or dumbbell incorporation, and working up to barbell introduction. The timeline for equipment progression will be dependent upon the postpartum woman's lifting experience, comfort level in using each type of equipment, and overall recovery process. If she is breastfeeding, relaxin levels will remain elevated and can cause ligament laxity and possibly pelvic or SIJ pain even if she is an experienced weight lifter [51].

Equipment selection and weight lifted will have a significant impact on prolapse. Women who return to strenuous lifting too soon postpartum can be at an increased risk for developing prolapse [2]. Women with prolapse can still lift lighter loads if they are able to properly manage intra abdominal pressure and are not bearing down into the pelvic floor while lifting. Bearing down into the pelvic floor while lifting is an inappropriate but common strategy for attempting to stabilize the pelvis when there is a lack of strength or function in the core. Addressing diastasis recti if present will also encourage proper intra abdominal pressure management and provide strength and function to the core and pelvis and limit the need for other compensatory movements and strategies that can lead to prolapse.

Jumping and plyometrics are some of the last impact exercises that are introduced in postpartum exercise plans. High impact exercises such as jumping and plyometrics can reveal pelvic dysfunction in the form of urinary incontinence. Because these exercises place a high level of stress on the pelvic floor, postpartum women who had not experienced urinary incontinence before may experience it for the first time while attempting jumping or plyometrics [2]. Urinary incontinence should be recognized as a symptom of pelvic floor dysfunction and a referral to a pelvic floor therapist should be recommended. It is also a sign that the pelvic floor is not ready for such high impact and scaling back may be necessary.

To date, there is no evidence to support a definitive intensity maximum after the 13 week postpartum period without any RPE or heart rate restrictions outside of normal, age-appropriate ranges. The ACSM does suggest that training volume should progress gradually at 2–10% per week in direct relation to postpartum recovery progress and goals of the postpartum woman [2].

## 7. Conclusion

Considering all components of pregnancy and postpartum recovery is essential to planning and implementing resistance training into an exercise program. When done correctly, resistance training can be a safe form of exercise for pregnant and postpartum women and can enhance their pregnancy, supplement their postpartum recovery, and add to their quality of life.

## Author details

Aly Matejka
University of Findlay, Findlay, Ohio, United States

*Address all correspondence to: alymatejka@gmail.com

## References

[1] Santo E, Forbes P, Oken E, Belfort M. Detriments of physical activity frequency and provider advice during pregnancy. BMC Pregnancy and Childbirth. 2017;**17**:286. DOI: 10.1186/s12884-017-1460-z

[2] Selman R et al. Maximizing recovery in the postpartum period: A timeline for rehabilitation from pregnancy through return to sport. IJSPT. 2022;**17**(6):1170-1183. DOI: 10.26603/001c.37863

[3] Menke et al. Physical activity during pregnancy and newborn body composition: A systematic review. International Journal of Environmental Research and Public Health. 2022;**19**:7127. DOI: 10.3390/ijerph19127127

[4] Prewitt-White T et al. Breaking barriers: Women's experiences of crossfit training during pregnancy. Women in Sport and Physical Activity Journal. 2018;**26**:33-42. DOI: 10.1123/wspaj.2017-0024

[5] Budler L, Budler M. Physical activity during pregnancy: A systematic review for the assessment of current evidence with future recommendations. BMC Sports Science, Medicine and Rehabilitation. 2022;**14**(1):133. DOI: 10.1186/s13102-022-00524-z

[6] Sanbria-Martinez G et al. Effectiveness of physical activity interventions on preventing gestational diabetes mellitus and excessive maternal weight gain: A meta-analysis. BJOG: An International Journal of Obstetrics and Gynaecology. 2015;**122**(9):1167-1174. DOI: 10.1111/1471-0528.13429

[7] Ajibua A et al. Exercise prescription for stages of pregnancy and postpartum period. JERP. 2021;**2**(2):40-50. DOI: 10.53016/jerp.v2i2.15

[8] Blotta R et al. Collagen I and III in women with diastasis recti. Clinics (São Paulo, Brazil). 2018;**7**(73):319. DOI: 10.6061/clinics/2018/e319

[9] Olson D et al. Exercise in pregnancy. Current Sports Medicine Reports. 2009;**8**(3):147-153. DOI: 10.1249/JSR.0b013e3181a61d51

[10] White E et al. Motives for and barriers to exercising across trimesters of pregnancy in health club members. Human Movement. 2020;**21**(3):21-30. DOI: 10.5114/hm.2020.91342

[11] Ritacco C et al. Muscle strengthening exercises during pregnancy are associated with increased energy and reduced fatigue. Journal of Psychosomatic Obstetrics and Gynaecology. 2016;**37**(2):68-72. DOI: 10.3109/0167482X.2016.1155552

[12] White E et al. Resistance training during pregnancy and perinatal outcomes. Journal of Physical Activity & Health. 2014;**11**(6):1141-1148. DOI: 10.1123/jpah.2012-0350

[13] Yaping X et al. A meta-analysis of the effects of resistance training on blood sugar and pregnancy outcomes. Midwifery. 2020:91, 102839. DOI: 10.1016/j.midw.2020.102839

[14] Keating N et al. Aerobic or resistance exercise for improved glycaemic control and pregnancy outcomes in women with gestational diabetes mellitus: A systematic review. International Journal of Environmental Research and Public Health. 2022;**19**(17):10791. DOI: 10.3390/ijerph191710791

[15] Eiland E et al. Preeclampsia 2012. Journal of Pregnancy. 2012;**2012**:586578. DOI: 10.1155/2012/586578

[16] Sperstad J et al. Diastasis recti abdominis during pregnancy and 12 months after childbirth: Prevalence, risk factors and report of lumbopelvic pain. British Journal of Sports Medicine. 2016;**50**(17):1092-1096. DOI: 10.1136/bjsports-2016-096065

[17] Laframboise F et al. Postpartum exercise intervention targeting diastasis recti abdominis. International Journal of Exercise Science. 2021;**14**(3):400-409

[18] Morino S et al. Pelvic alignment changes during the perinatal period. PLoS One. 2019;**14**(10):e0223776. DOI: 10.1371/journal.pone.0223776

[19] Michalska A et al. Diastasis recti abdominis—A review of treatment methods. Ginekologia Polska. 2018;**89**(2):97-101. DOI: 10.5603/GP.a2018.0016

[20] Doshani A et al. Uterine prolapse. BMJ. 2007;**335**(7624):819-823. DOI: 10.1136/bmj.39356.604074.BE

[21] Humphries A et al. The collateral venous system in late pregnancy: A systematic review of the literature. Clinical Anatomy. 2017;**30**(8):1087-1095. DOI: 10.1002/ca.22959

[22] Humphries A et al. The effect of supine positioning on maternal hemodynamics during late pregnancy. The Journal of Maternal-Fetal & Neonatal Medicine. 2019;**32**(23):3923-3930. DOI: 10.1080/14767058.2018.1478958

[23] Weintraub A et al. Narrative review of the epidemiology, diagnosis and pathophysiology of pelvic organ prolapse. IBJU. 2020;**46**(1):5-14. DOI: 10.1590/S1677-5538.IBJU.2018.0581

[24] Patel K et al. Natural history of urinary incontinence from first childbirth to 30-months postpartum. Archives of Gynecology and Obstetrics. 2021;**304**(3):713-724. DOI: 10.1007/s00404-021-06134-3

[25] Aldabe D et al. Pregnancy-related pelvic girdle pain and its relationship with relaxin levels during pregnancy: A systematic review. European Spine Journal. 2012;**21**(9):1769-1776. DOI: 10.1007/s00586-012-2162-x

[26] Bani D. Relaxin: A pleiotropic hormone. General Pharmacology. 1997;**28**(1):13-22. DOI: 10.1016/s0306-3623(96)00171-1

[27] Robinson H et al. Pelvic girdle pain-associations between risk factors in early pregnancy and disability or pain intensity in late pregnancy: A prospective cohort study. BMC Musculoskeletal Disorders. 2010;**11**:91. DOI: 10.1186/1471-2474-11-91

[28] Olsen M et al. Evaluation of self-administered tests for pelvic girdle pain in pregnancy. BMC Musculoskeletal Disorders. 2014;**15**:138. DOI: 10.1186/1471-2474-15-138

[29] O'Connor P et al. Safety and efficacy of supervised strength training adopted in pregnancy. Journal of Physical Activity & Health. 2011;**8**(3):309-320. DOI: 10.1123/jpah.8.3.309

[30] Artal R, Toole M. Guidelines of the American College of Obstetricians and Gynecologists for exercise during pregnancy and the postpartum period. British Journal of Sports Medicine. 2003;**37**(1):6-12. DOI: 10.1136/bjsm.37.1.6

[31] Oostdam N et al. Design of FitFor2 study: The effects of an exercise program on insulin sensitivity and plasma glucose levels in pregnant women at high risk for gestational diabetes. BMC Pregnancy and Childbirth. 2009;**9**:1. DOI: 10.1186/1471-2393-9-1

[32] Wing C et al. Pregnancy and exercise guidelines—Fifty years makes a difference. ACSM's Health & Fitness Journal. 2016;**20**(2):4-6. DOI: 10.1249/FIT.0000000000000183

[33] Gould S et al. Resistance training does not decrease placental blood flow during valsalva maneuver: A novel use of 3d doppler power flow ultrasonography. Sports Health. 2021;**13**(5):476-481. DOI: 10.1177/19417381211000717

[34] Sze E et al. Pregnancy, labor, delivery, and pelvic organ prolapse. Obstetrics and Gynecology. 2002;**100** (5 Pt 1):981-986. DOI: 10.1016/s0029-7844(02)02246-9

[35] Smith L et al. Incidence of and risk factors for perineal trauma: A prospective observational study. BMC Pregnancy and Childbirth. 2013;**13**:59. DOI: 10.1186/1471-2393-13-59

[36] Rikard-Bell J et al. Perineal outcome and the risk of pelvic floor dysfunction: A cohort study of primiparous women. The Australian & New Zealand Journal of Obstetrics & Gynaecology. 2014;**54**(4): 371-376. DOI: 10.1111/ajo.12222

[37] Sung S, Mahdy H. Cesarean Section. Treasure Island, FL: StatPearls Publishing; 2022. DOI: NBK546707

[38] Liang C et al. Correlation of pelvic organ prolapse quantification system scores with obstetric parameters and lower urinary tract symptoms in primiparae postpartum. International Urogynecology Journal and Pelvic Floor Dysfunction. 2007;**18**(5):537-541. DOI: 10.1007/s00192-006-0195-6

[39] Campeau L et al. Pelvic floor disorders: Linking genetic risk factors to biochemical changes. BJUI. 2011;**108**(8):1240-1247. DOI: 10.1111/j.1464-410X.2011.10385.x

[40] Behnke A. The physical and emotional effects of postpartum hormone levels. International Journal of Childbirth. 2003;**18**(2):11-14. Available from: http://www.encognitive.com/files/The%20Physical%20and%20Emotional%20Effects%20of%20Postpartum%20Hormone%20Levels_0.pdf

[41] Meek J et al. Policy statement: Breastfeeding and the use of human milk. Pediatrics. 2022;**150**(1):e2022057988. DOI: 10.1542/peds.2022-057988

[42] Horng H et al. Estrogen effects on wound healing. International Journal of Molecular Sciences. 2017;**18**(11):2325. DOI: 10.3390/ijms18112325

[43] Parul et al. Impact of diastasis recti abdominis muscle on the posture and quality of like in the primiparous postpartum women a cross sectional survey. Indian Journal of Medical Sciences. 2021;**8**:24. DOI: 2394-2800

[44] Thomas K, Foreman S. Infant sleep and feeding pattern: Effects on maternal sleep. JMWH. 2005;**50**(5):399-404. DOI: 10.1016/j.jmwh.2005.04.010

[45] Hunter L et al. A selective review of maternal sleep characteristics in the postpartum period. Journal of Obstetric, Gynecologic, and Neonatal Nursing. 2009;**38**(1):60-68. DOI: 10.1111/j.1552-6909.2008.00309.x

[46] Hendrick V et al. Hormonal changes in the postpartum and implications for postpartum depression. Psychosomatics. 1998;**39**(2):93-101. DOI: 10.1016/S0033-3182(98)71355-6

[47] Miller L. Postpartum depression. Journal of the American Medical Association. 2002;**287**(6):762-765. DOI: 10.1001/jama.287.6.762

[48] Postnatal exercise guidelines. Freshly centered. The Interne 2019.

Available from: http://freshlycentered.com/2019/12/_trashed/ [Accessed: October 10, 2019]

[49] Pereira L, et al. Are transversus abdominis/oblique internal and pelvic floor muscles coactivated during pregnancy and postpartum? Neurourology and Urodynamics. 2013;**32**(5):416-419. DOI: 10.1002/nau.22315

[50] Ainscough-Potts A et al. The response of the transverse abdominis and internal oblique muscles to different postures. Manual Therapy. 2006;**11**(1):54-60. DOI: 10.1016/j.math.2005.03.007

[51] Relaxin. Cleveland Clinic. [Internet]. 2022. Available from: https://my.clevelandclinic.org/health/body/24305-relaxin [Accessed: October 15, 2022]

Section 3

# Ageing

## Chapter 6

# Strength Training, Quality of Life, and Health in Elderly

*Francisco Saavedra*

## Abstract

The normal aging process is characterized by a progression of physiological events throughout the life cycle. Age-related changes take place throughout the body and are most prominent in later years. The aims and purposes of this study were to: i) provide a summary of existing and relevant research, ii) assess exercise program variables, and iii) give practical evidence-based recommendations for exercise prescription and resistance training in older adults, according to international guidelines. Using an evidence-based approach, we combined scientific data, experts' statements and end-user concerns to improve references for the aging population's interests, values, requirements, and choices. Thus, the position statement assesses the main studies obtained after a thorough analysis of the literature. In conclusion, we highlight that strength training alone or combined with aerobic training is a fundamental part of the primary prevention of many chronic diseases in older adults, in addition to delaying the progression and reducing the symptoms of related chronic conditions. Multicomponent exercise programs, especially strength exercises that include muscle power training, are the most effective interventions for buffering the impact of physical disability and other adverse health-related outcomes, even in the oldest old.

**Keywords:** aging, physical activity, strength, wellbeing, health-related outcomes

## 1. Introduction

Older adults are the fastest-growing age group. Physiological changes associated with primary aging and concurrent chronic diseases have an adverse impact on functional capacity, health outcomes, and quality of life [1]. The normal aging process is characterized by a progression of physiological events that occur throughout the life cycle. Age-related changes take place throughout the body and are most prominent in later years.

Advanced age, even if not associated with the development of a serious chronic disease, is accompanied by a multiplicity of biological modifications that may contribute to reducing skeletal muscle mass, strength, and function, leading to an overall decline in physiological resilience (capacity to withstand and recover from stressors). It is also related to reduced muscle size (muscle atrophy), motor unit loss, and a decrease in contraction speed, which in turn lead to lower muscle strength, power, and resistance [2–4].



IntechOpen

As a multifaceted and complex phenomenon, aging manifests itself differently among individuals during their lifetime and is conditional on interactions between genetic, environmental, behavioral, and demographic characteristics [5]. The literature reports that sarcopenia affects motor and muscle performance [3, 6–8]. Losses in muscle function can reduce physical fitness and independence in the activities of daily living. Moreover, significant dependence levels of older people are positively associated with greater fear and risk of falling and lower quality of life [9].

Since most of the risk factors are associated with an increase in chronic diseases with (advanced) age, regular physical activity is essential to attenuate the functional declines associated with aging and improve physical and psychological health-related outcomes among older adults [1, 10].

As such, and considering that much of the senior population is sedentary with low levels of physical fitness, thc aims and purposes of this study were to: (i) provide a summary of existing and relevant research, (ii) assess exercise program variables, and (iii) give practical evidence-based recommendations for exercise prescription and resistance training in older adults, according to international guidelines.

## 2. Process

Using an evidence-based approach, we combined scientific data, experts' statements, and end-user concerns to improve references for the interests, values, requirements, and choices of the aging population. Thus, the position statement presents an assessment of the main studies obtained after a thorough analysis of the literature.

Since there is a wide-ranging biological dissimilarity among elders of related age, and developmental modifications in voluntary muscle usually start in adulthood, no typical designation of the senior period based on chronological age remained considered adequate. In its place, due to the wide physiological and functional variety, and the beginning of age-related consequences for voluntary muscles, studies involving subjects aged 50 years and older were analyzed.

## 3. Evidence for summary statements

Resistance training is the most effective method for maintaining and increasing lean body mass and improving muscle strength and endurance [11]. It is recommended as part of the physical activity guidelines that include working all major muscle groups two or more days a week [10, 12]. Older adults can reap numerous health benefits from resistance training, such as increased muscle strength and mass in addition to maintaining bone density. Furthermore, certain dimensions of health-related quality of life have been shown to improve in older adults as a result of resistance training [13].

Given the adverse physical, social, and emotional consequences of aging, prevention and treatment strategies are essential for the health and well-being of older adults [5, 10, 13]. Among the contributors to the aging process, muscle disuse is an avoidable and changeable factor. Strength exercise is a significant component of a comprehensive workout plan to balance the widely recognized constructive effects of aerobic exercise on well-being and physical abilities [12]. There is vigorous and compelling evidence that strength training can buffer the consequences of aging on the neuromuscular role and functional aptitude [12–17]. Different procedures of strength training can potentially increase muscle strength, mass, and power output [12]. Moreover, available evidence reveals a dose–response association, where volume and intensity are strongly related to adaptations to resistance exercise [14, 18].

With this in mind, different institutions suggest that adults should engage in moderate- to high-intensity muscle-strengthening activities including working all major muscle groups two or more days a week [10, 12]. For aging adults, the same muscle-strengthening guidelines apply, since resistance training may promote even greater benefits for this population. Several health problems affecting older adults can be mitigated or even prevented through a regular resistance training program [13]. For example, older people have a greater risk of premature death due to falls, which in turn are associated with age-related declines in muscle fitness and balance that may be reduced/improved via different forms of resistance training [19–22].

Seniors can obtain several additional health paybacks from strength preparation, furthermore, greater muscle area and power [13, 23]. Findings have shown that

| Variable | Resistance exercise |
|---|---|
| Bone mineral density | ↑↑ |
| Risk of falls | ↓ |
| Osteoarthritis | ↓ |
| % fat | ↓ |
| LBM | ↑↑ |
| Strength | ↑↑↑ |
| Local muscle endurance | ↑↑↑ |
| Glucose metabolism | |
| Insulin response to glucose challenge | ↓↓ |
| Basal insulin levels | ↓ |
| Insulin sensitivity | ↑↑ |
| Serum lipids | |
| HDL | ↑↔ |
| LDL | ↓↔ |
| Resting heart rate | ↔ |
| Stroke volume | ↔ |
| Blood pressure at rest | |
| Systolic | ↔ |
| Diastolic | ↓↔ |
| $VO_{2max}$ | ↑ |
| Endurance time | ↑↑ |
| Physical function | ↑↑↑ |
| Independent living/mobility | ↑↑↑ |
| Basal metabolism | ↑↑ |

*Adapted from Pollock and Vincent [32].*

**Table 1.**
*Effects of resistance training on health and fitness variables.*

strength training can improve bone mineral density [24, 25], lipoprotein profiles [26], glycemic control [27], body composition [28], symptoms of frailty [29], metabolic syndrome risk factors [30], and cardiovascular disease markers [31]. This cumulative aggregate of evidence has provided additional support for the findings initially reported in the seminal review by Pollock and Vincent ([32], see **Table 1**), demonstrating that resistance training plays a significant role in improving numerous health factors associated with the prevention of chronic diseases throughout life.

Taken as a whole, evidence indicates that resistance training improves physical health, functional ability, and quality of life in older persons, even in the presence of frailty and chronic illness. Moreover, resistance training levels in line with international guidelines have been associated with increased physical fitness, better cardiovascular risk profile, and decreased overall (all-cause) mortality [33–35].

According to Hunter et al. [36], a substantial portion of the reductions in age-related strength and muscle function is mediated by decreases in daily physical activity, which in turn induce greater sarcopenia. This results in a positive feedback loop that worsens over time (**Figure 1**). Thus, interrupting this cycle is of paramount importance to maintain the functional capacity and quality of life of aging adults.

All resistance exercise programs should match the individual needs and competencies of older adults. A thorough medical/physical evaluation should be performed to rule out possible comorbidities and contraindications to physical exercise (myocardial infarction, or unstable angina, uncontrolled hypertension, acute heart failure, and complete venous arterial blockage).

Moreover, the established plan/program and its potential side effects (muscle injury, joint injury, and fractures) should also be monitored. In short, exercise prescription should be specific, individualized (health status, chronic disease risk factors, behavioral characteristics, personal goals, and exercise preferences), and progressive to optimize and maximize the magnitude of the strength adaptations in older adults [37–39].

Nonetheless, resistance training may also be prescribed concurrently with aerobic training since both types of physical exercise produce distinct benefits, such as improvements in neuromuscular and cardiovascular functions [16], respectively, and because both muscle strength and aerobic fitness are inversely associated with

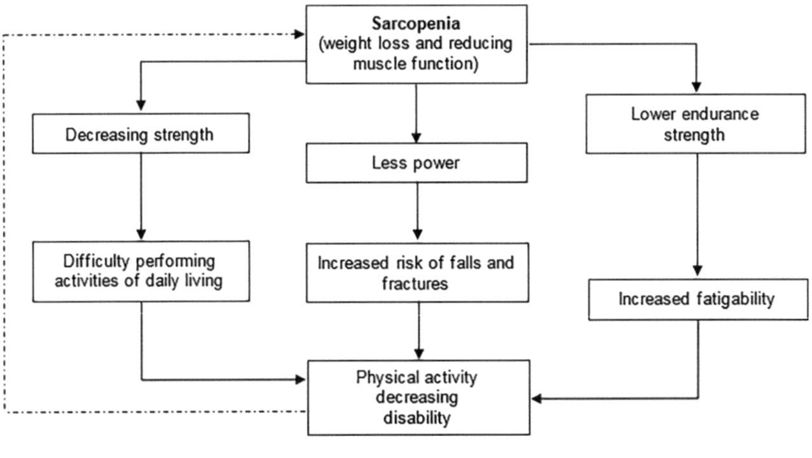


**Figure 1.**
*Model of age-related functional changes in sarcopenia (adapted from Hunter et al. [36]).*

| Organization | Type | Mode | Duration | Intensity | Frequency |
|---|---|---|---|---|---|
| *American College of Sport Medicine* [40] | Aerobic | Rapid Walking | 75'–150' week | Moderate to Vigorous | Minimum 3 days/week |
| | Resistance Training | 8–10 exercises 3–4 sets 8–12 reps. | | 75% de 1RM | Minimum 2 days/week |
| | Flexibility | Complementary to other types of exercise (static and dynamic; major muscle groups) | | | |
| *American Heart Association* [41] | Aerobic | Walking | 150' week | Moderate | 3 – 7 days/week |
| | | Rapid Walking | 90' week | Vigorous | 2 days/week |
| | Resistance Training | 2–4 sets 8–12 reps. | | 75% de 1RM | 3 days/week |

*RM: Repetition Maximum; Reps: Repetitions.*

**Table 2.**
*International recommendations of multicomponent physical activity for healthy adults.*

all-cause mortality in older individuals [12, 37–39]. With this in mind, different international institutions have suggested exercise guidelines and recommendations that involve a combination of aerobic and resistance training, agility/balance, and static and dynamic flexibility exercises for adults [40–42] (see **Table 2**).

To promote and maintain health, all healthy adults need to accumulate at least 150 minutes/week of moderate-intensity aerobic exercise (60–70% of maximum heart rate, or 12–13 on a perceived exertion scale range of 6–20 points), on most days of the week or at least 75 minutes of vigorous aerobic activity (70–90% of maximum heart rate, or 14 to 16 on a perceived exertion scale variety of 6 to 20 points). Adults must still execute activities that preserve or rise muscle power, at minimum two non-consecutive days per week. In addition to the minimum levels of aerobic and resistance exercise recommended for adults, older people are advised to perform stretching and balance exercises at least 2 to 3 times/week to prevent falling and maintain and improve their autonomy and quality of life [12, 38–43].

Resistance exercise must be performed 2 to 3 times a week, using 3 sets of 8–12 repetitions, with an initial intensity of 20–30% of 1RM, developing to 70% of 1RM. Strength training can be performed using resistance machines that work major muscle groups (e.g., leg press and knee extension).

Nevertheless, movements that involve monoarticular actions have a minor cardiovascular answer (increased heart rate and blood pressure) but, at the start of the training procedure, are more appropriate to use in persons with cardiovascular disease [38–40]. To enhance the development of functional capability in aging adults, the resistance training program should also include strength exercises that reproduce the activities of quotidian living, such as rising and sitting [44].

Muscle power (high-speed) training may be more beneficial in terms of functional improvement than a muscle endurance training program (low speed) [45].

This type of training, with light loads and explosive movements, should be included in the activities prescribed to older adults because it may be associated with an improved functional capacity [38, 39, 45]. Cardiovascular endurance training should include sets of walking in different directions and speeds, walking on a treadmill, and walking up and downstairs. This activity should last 5–10 minutes in the first weeks, progressing to 15–30 minutes [46].

| Benefits | Modality | Prescription |
|---|---|---|
| Improved cardiovascular endurance | Walking Cycling | 60–80% HRmax (40–60% $VO_2$max) 5–30 min/session 3 days/week |
| Improved muscle mass and strength | Free weights Variable resistance machines | 8–10 reps/set (20RM) 4–6 reps/set (15RM) 6–8 exercises large muscle groups |
| Power and Functional Capacity | Exercises of daily living (rising/sitting and climbing up and downstairs) Power exercises (high speed/mild to moderate load) | 8–10 reps/set 2–3 Sets (60% 1RM) with the maximum possible speed |
| Flexibility | Stretches Yoga/Pilates | 10–15 min 2–3 days/week |
| Balance | Exercises in tandem and semi-tandem position, multidirectional movement with extra weight (2–4 kg), heel-toe walking, climbing stairs with assistance, transfer of body weight (from one leg to the other) and modified Tai Chi exercises | Daily sessions |

*HR: Heart Rate; RM: Repetition Maximum; Reps: Repetitions.*

**Table 3.**
*Guidelines for exercise prescription in older adults (adapted from Casas Herrero et al. [40]).*

Balance training should include exercises in the tandem and semi-tandem position, multidirectional movements under load (2–4 kg), heel-toe walking, climbing stairs with assistance, and body mass transfer (from one leg to the other). Modified tai chi exercises, yoga, stretching, and balance training may also improve physical functioning and benefit patients with hypertension, heart disease, and arthritis (**Table 3**) [16–25].

Multicomponent training programs should include gradual increases in the volume, intensity, and complexity of cardiovascular, strength, and balance exercises. Alternate training days of muscle strength and cardiovascular endurance exercises are an excellent stimulus for improving strength, power, and cardiovascular resistance. When performing training programs that combine strength and cardiovascular endurance, one should preferably perform strength before cardio training [39]. In individuals with low physical fitness levels and/or without regular exercise habits, applying a low training volume may facilitate adherence to the program [12].

## 4. Evidence for summary statements

Strength training alone, or combined with aerobic training, is a fundamental part of the primary prevention of many chronic diseases in older adults, in addition to delaying the progression and reducing the symptoms of related chronic conditions. Most of the benefits occur with at least 150 minutes of moderate physical exercise a week. Vigorous aerobic and strength exercises are recommended at least 2 days/week.

Multicomponent exercise programs, especially strength exercises that include muscle power training, are the most effective interventions for buffering the impact of physical disability and other adverse health-related outcomes, even in the oldest old. These programs are also valuable interventions in other frailty domains, such as falls and cognitive decline.

Physical exercise and strength training should be adapted to the characteristics and contraindications of each individual, and prescribed with a progressive individualized plan, to produce continued benefits, like any other medical treatment.

Strength training should also be tailored to match functional needs and preferences, based on a pragmatic strategy that makes exercise both sustainable and safe. Such a strategy incorporates motivational elements and knowledge/monitoring of achievable benefits using an idiographic approach.

## Conflict of interest

The authors declare no conflict of interest.

## Author details

Francisco Saavedra[1,2]

1 University of Trás-os-Montes and Alto Douro (UTAD), Vila Real, Portugal

2 Research Centre in Sports Sciences, Health Sciences and Human Development (CIDESD), UTAD, Vila Real, Portugal

*Address all correspondence to: fjfsaave@utad.pt

## References


[1] Zaleski AL, Taylor BA, Panza GA, Wu Y, Pescatello LS, Thompson PD, et al. Coming of age: Considerations in the prescription of exercise for older adults. Methodist DeBakey Cardiovascular Journal. 2016;**12**(2):98-104. DOI: 10.14797/mdcj-12-2-98

[2] Arakelian VM, Goulart CDL, Mendes RG, Sousa NM, Trimer R, Guizilini S, et al. Physiological responses in different intensities of resistance exercise - Critical load and the effects of aging process. Journal of Sports Sciences. 2019;**37**(12):1420-1428. DOI: 10.1080/02640414.2018.1561389

[3] Frontera WR, Hughes VA, Fielding RA, Fiatarone MA, Evans WJ, Roubenoff R. Aging of skeletal muscle: A 12-yr longitudinal study. Journal of Applied Physiology. 1985/2000;**88**(4):1321-1326. DOI: 10.1152/jappl.2000.88.4.1321

[4] Traczyk A, Kuźba K, Chłystek J, Potyra K, Abramczyk A, Łakomski M. Resistance training for the elderly. Review of the literature. Journal of Education, Health and Sport. 2018;**8**(9):1048-1057

[5] Ben-Shlomo Y, Cooper R, Kuh D. The last two decades of life course epidemiology, and its relevance for research on ageing. International Journal of Epidemiology. 2016;**45**(4):973-988. DOI: 10.1093/ije/dyw096

[6] Greenlund LJ, Nair KS. Sarcopenia-consequences, mechanisms, and potential therapies. Mechanisms of Ageing and Development. 2003;**124**(3):287-299. DOI: 10.1016/s0047-6374(02)00196-3

[7] Moran J, Ramirez-Campillo R, Granacher U. Effects of jumping exercise on muscular power in older adults: A meta-analysis. Sports Medicine. 2018;**48**(12):2843-2857. DOI: 10.1007/s40279-018-1002-5

[8] Vandervoort AA. Aging of the human neuromuscular system. Muscle & Nerve. 2002;**25**(1):17-25. DOI: 10.1002/mus.1215

[9] Carrasco-Poyatos M, Rubio-Arias JA, Ballesta-García I, Ramos-Campo DJ. Pilates vs. muscular training in older women. Effects in functional factors and the cognitive interaction: A randomized controlled trial. Physiology & Behavior. 2019;**201**:157-164. DOI: 10.1016/j.physbeh.2018.12.008

[10] American College of Sports Medicine, Chodzko-Zajko WJ, Proctor DN, et al. American College of sports medicine position stand. Exercise and physical activity for older adults. Medicine and Science in Sports and Exercise. 2009;**41**(7):1510-1530

[11] Hass CJ, Feigenbaum MS, Franklin BA. Prescription of resistance training for healthy populations. Sports Medicine. 2001;**31**(14):953-964. DOI:10.2165/00007256-200131140-00001

[12] Fragala MS, Cadore EL, Dorgo S, Izquierdo M, Kraemer WJ, Peterson MD, et al. Resistance training for older adults: Position statement from the national strength and conditioning association. Journal of Strength and Conditioning Research. 2019;**33**(8):2019-2052. DOI: 10.1519/JSC.0000000000003230

[13] Hart P, Buck DJ. The effect of resistance training on health-related quality of life in older adults: Systematic review and meta-analysis. Health Promotion Perspective. 2019;**9**(1):1-12. DOI: 10.15171/hpp.2019.01

[14] Borde R, Hortobágyi T, Granacher U. Dose-response relationships of resistance training in healthy old adults: A systematic review and meta-analysis. Sports Medicine. 2015;**45**(12):1693-1720. DOI: 10.1007/s40279-015-0385-9

[15] Cadore EL, Casas-Herrero A, Zambom-Ferraresi F, Idoate F, Millor N, Gómez M, et al. Multicomponent exercises including muscle power training enhance muscle mass, power output, and functional outcomes in institutionalized frail nonagenarians. Age, (Dordr). 2014;**36**(2):773-785. DOI: 10.1007/s11357-013-9586-z

[16] Cadore EL, Izquierdo M, Pinto SS, Alberton CL, Pinto RS, Baroni BM, et al. Neuromuscular adaptations to concurrent training in the elderly: Effects of intrasession exercise sequence. Age, (Dordr). 2013;**35**(3):891-803. DOI: 10.1007/s11357-012-9405-y

[17] Silva RB, Eslick GD, Duque G. Exercise for falls and fracture prevention in long term care facilities: A systematic review and meta-analysis. Journal of the American Medical Directors Association. 2013;**14**(9):685-9.e2. DOI: 10.1016/j.jamda.2013.05.015

[18] Steib S, Schoene D, Pfeifer K. Dose-response relationship of resistance training in older adults: A meta-analysis. Medicine and Science in Sports and Exercise. 2010;**42**(5):902-914. DOI: 10.1249/MSS.0b013e3181c34465

[19] Bergen G, Stevens MR, Burns ER. Falls and fall injuries among adults aged ≥65 years - United States, 2014. MMWR. Morbidity and Mortality Weekly Report. 2016;**65**(37):993-998. DOI: 10.15585/mmwr.mm6537a2

[20] Ahmadiahangar A, Javadian Y, Babaei M, Heidari B, Hosseini SR, Aminzadeh M. The role of quadriceps muscle strength in the development of falls in the elderly people, a cross-sectional study. Chiropractic and Manual Therapies. 2018;**26**(1):1-6. DOI: 10.1186/s12998-018-0195-x

[21] Van Ancum JM, Pijnappels M, Jonkman NH, Scheerman K, Verlaan S, Meskers CGM, et al. Muscle mass and muscle strength are associated with pre-and post-hospitalization falls in older male inpatients: A longitudinal cohort study. BMC Geriatrics. 2018;**18**(1):116. DOI: 10.1186/s12877-018-0812-5

[22] Skinner EH, Dinh T, Hewitt M, Piper R, Thwaites C. An Ai Chi-based aquatic group improves balance and reduces falls in community-dwelling adults: A pilot observational cohort study. Physiotherapy Theory and Practice. 2016;**32**(8):581-590. DOI: 10.1080/09593985.2016.1227411

[23] Westcott WL. Resistance training is medicine: Effects of strength training on health. Current Sports Medicine Reports. 2012;**11**(4):209-216. DOI: 10.1249/JSR.0b013e31825dabb8

[24] Huovinen V, Ivaska KK, Kiviranta R, Bucci M, Lipponen H, Sandboge S, et al. Bone mineral density is increased after a 16-week resistance training intervention in elderly women with decreased muscle strength. European Journal of Endocrinology. 2016;**175**(6):571-582. DOI: 10.1530/EJE-16-0521

[25] Anek A, Kanungsukasem V, Bunyaratavej N. Effects of aerobic step combined with resistance training on biochemical bone markers, health-related physical fitness and balance in working women. Journal of the Medical Association of Thailand. 2015;**98**(Suppl. 8):S42-S51

[26] Ribeiro AS, Tomeleri CM, Souza MF, Pina FL, Schoenfeld BJ, Nascimento MA,

et al. Effect of resistance training on C-reactive protein, blood glucose and lipid profile in older women with differing levels of RT experience. Age, (Dordr). 2015;**37**(6):109. DOI: 10.1007/s11357-015-9849-y

[27] Takenami E, Iwamoto S, Shiraishi N, Kato A, Watanabe Y, Yamada Y, et al. Effects of low-intensity resistance training on muscular function and glycemic control in older adults with type 2 diabetes. Journal of Diabetes Investigation. 2019;**10**(2):331-338. DOI: 10.1111/jdi.12926

[28] Cavalcante EF, Ribeiro AS, do Nascimento MA, Silva AM, Tomeleri CM, Nabuco HCG, et al. Effects of different resistance training frequencies on fat in overweight/obese older women. International Journal of Sports Medicine. 2018;**39**(7):527-534. DOI: 10.1055/a-0599-6555

[29] Nagai K, Miyamato T, Okamae A, Tamaki A, Fujioka H, Wada Y, et al. Physical activity combined with resistance training reduces symptoms of frailty in older adults: A randomized controlled trial. Archives of Gerontology and Geriatrics. 2018;**76**:41-47. DOI: 10.1016/j.archger.2018.02.005

[30] Tomeleri CM, Souza MF, Burini RC, Cavaglieri CR, Ribeiro AS, Antunes M, et al. Resistance training reduces metabolic syndrome and inflammatory markers in older women: A randomized controlled trial. Journal of Diabetes. 2018;**10**(4):328-337. DOI: 10.1111/1753-0407.12614

[31] Shaw BS, Gouveia M, McIntyre S, Shaw I. Anthropometric and cardiovascular responses to hypertrophic resistance training in postmenopausal women. Menopause. 2016;**23**(11):1176-1181. DOI: 10.1097/gme.0000000000000687

[32] Pollock ML, Vincent KR. Resistance training for health. The President's council on physical fitness and sports research digest. 1996. Available from: http://fitness.foundation/s/Digest-1996_Resistance-Training-for-Health_Series-2-Number-8-December.pdf.

[33] Kamada M, Shiroma EJ, Buring JE, Miyachi M, Lee IM. Strength training and all-cause, cardiovascular disease, and cancer mortality in older women: A cohort study. Journal of the American Heart Association. 2017;**6**(11):e007677. DOI: 10.1161/jaha.117.007677

[34] Kraschnewski JL, Sciamanna CN, Poger JM, Rovniak LS, Lehman EB, Cooper AB, et al. Is strength training associated with mortality benefits? A 15-year cohort study of US older adults. Preventive Medicine. 2016;**87**:121-127. DOI: 10.1016/j.ypmed.2016.02.038

[35] Mernitz H, McDermott AY. Exercise and the elderly: A scientific rationale for exercise prescription. Journal of Clinical Outcomes Management. 2004;**11**(2):106-116

[36] Hunter GR, McCarthy JP, Bamman MM. Effects of resistance training on older adults. Sports Medicine. 2004;**34**(5):329-348. DOI: 10.2165/00007256-200434050-00005

[37] Haff G, Triplett NT. Essentials of Strength Training and Conditioning. 4th ed. Champaign, IL: Human Kinetics; 2016. p. 462

[38] Cadore EL, Rodríguez-Mañas L, Sinclair A, Izquierdo M. Effects of different exercise interventions on risk of falls, gait ability, and balance in physically frail older adults: A systematic review. Rejuvenation Research. 2013;**16**(2):105-114. DOI: 10.1089/rej.2012.1397

[39] Cadore EL, Izquierdo M. How to simultaneously optimize muscle strength, power, functional capacity, and cardiovascular gains in the elderly: An update. Age, (Dordr). 2013;**35**(6):2329-2344. DOI: 10.1007/s11357-012-9503-x

[40] Pescatello LS. ACSM's Guidelines for Exercise Testing and Prescription. 10th ed. Philadelphia: Wolters Kluwer/Lippincott Williams & Wilkins Health; 2017

[41] Riegel B, Moser DK, Buck HG, Dickson VV, Dunbar SB, Lee CS, et al. American heart association council on cardiovascular and stroke nursing; council on peripheral vascular disease; and council on quality of care and outcomes research. Self-care for the prevention and management of cardiovascular disease and stroke: A scientific statement for healthcare professionals from the American heart association. Journal of the American Heart Association. 2017;**6**(9):e006997. DOI: 10.1161/JAHA.117.006997

[42] American College of Sports Medicine. American College of Sports Medicine position stand. Progression models in resistance training for healthy adults. Medicine and Science in Sports and Exercise. 2009;**41**(3):687-608. DOI: 10.1249/MSS.0b013e3181915670

[43] Izquierdo M, Häkkinen K, Ibañez J, Garrues M, Antón A, Zúñiga A, et al. Effects of strength training on muscle power and serum hormonesin middle age and older men. Journal of Applied Physiology. 2001;**90**(4):1497-1507. DOI: 10.1152/jappl.2001.90.4.1497

[44] Casas Herrero Á, Cadore EL, Martínez Velilla N, Izquierdo Redin M. El ejercicio físico en el anciano frágil: una actualización [Physical exercise in the frail elderly: An update]. Revista Espanola de Geriatria y Gerontologia. 2015;**50**(2):74-81. DOI: 10.1016/j.regg.2014.07.003

[45] Izquierdo M, Cadore EL. Muscle power training in the institutionalized frail: A new approach to counteracting functional declines and very late-life disability. Current Medical Research and Opinion. 2014;**30**(7):1385-1390. DOI: 10.1185/03007995.2014.908175

[46] Cadore EL, Moneo AB, Mensat MM, Muñoz AR, Casas-Herrero A, Rodriguez-Mañas L, et al. Positive effects of resistance training in frail elderly patients with dementia after long-term physical restraint. Age, (Dordr). 2014;**36**(2):801-811. DOI: 10.1007/s11357-013-9599-7

Chapter 7

# Functional Capacity in Advanced Older Adults

*Abrão José Melhem Junior, Miguel Morita Fernandes-Silva and David Livingstone Alves Figueiredo*

## Abstract

Oldest-old adults are expected to represent 4.8% of the world population in 2030 (400 million). Aging influences functional capacity (FC), which is relevant information for this subpopulation and can be assessed by maximal oxygen uptake (VO2max) with a conventional exercise test (ET). Exercise-based programs for advanced older adults could improve health status and multiple studies support resistance training as an important option. An observational, retrospective study on FC assessment, with VO2max assessment, in the oldest-old adults, is presented. Eighty-six individuals, ≥75 years old, were included. FC was estimated by VO2max obtained with treadmill ET. Two groups with different FC were compared (A group: <24 mg/kg/min and B group: ≥24 mg/kg/min). Most important differences were found in body mass index and heart rate, with a correlation between these variables and both with VO2max. These findings can help the oldest-old adults' health care, once exercise programs provide multiple benefits for this subpopulation improving these specific variables, and other clinical aspects. Pre-participation assessment could promote safety, comfort, adherence, and effectiveness in advanced older adults. Exercise programs, including resistance training, impact quality of life, cognitive status, frailty symptoms, risk factors, and all-cause mortality.

**Keywords:** older adults, functional capacity, VO2max, exercise test, body mass index, heart rate

## 1. Introduction

Oldest-old adults may represent 5.5% of Brazilian population in 2030, about 12 million people; at the same time, the world is expected to achieve 400 million (4.8%) older adults with 75 years or more [1, 2]. Population aging is a worldwide concerning issue, as it is associated with the increasing prevalence of non-transmissible chronic diseases (NCD) and cardiovascular risk factors (RF); and the World Health Organization (WHO) adds the notion of functional capacity (FC) as a determinant of the degree of aging. FC varies among individuals, under genetic influences, but is also affected by social, cultural, environmental, and political issues. Determinants of the elderly's capacity are not only the progression of age but also choices, pathological processes, or interventions, at different times in the life. Then, another concept is presented: healthy or active aging, as the "process of development and maintenance of functional capacity that allows well-being in old age" [1]. Elderly-focused exercise programs, resistance training programs (RTP) included, aim to increase functionality, independence, and quality of life [3]. Functional increments have been related to lower cardiovascular and mortality risk rates in the elderly [4].

A paradox is that the growing oldest-old adult group is, unfortunately, less contemplated in elderly studies and, almost always, excluded in general population studies [5–7]. Several studies on obesity in the elderly found controversial results, with unfavorable [8], neutral [9] and favorable [10] results. The natural process of cardiovascular aging involves changes in structure and function that expose individuals to an exponential increase in the incidence and prevalence of cardiovascular diseases, such as coronary artery disease (CAD), heart failure (HF), atrial fibrillation (AF), and stroke [11]. Physical inactivity has been associated with being overweight, poor RF control, development of NCD, lower quality of life, and higher mortality in advanced elderly [12].

## 2. Functional capacity assessment

The evaluation of pathophysiological conditions, with emphasis on FC, could help in the inclusion, adherence, and safeguarding of resistance training programs (RTP) [13]. Many methods, such as questionnaires about activity or frailty [13], walking and movement tests [14], and tests with associated myocardial ischemia search [15] are useful in this assessment. FC can be affected by aging due to myocardial, blood vessels, and metabolic impairments in the presence or absence of detectable cardiovascular disease. The gold standard for FC assessment is the cardiopulmonary exercise test, with direct determination of maximum oxygen consumption (VO2max) [16, 17]. FC can also be assessed in advanced elderly with a safe, effective, and well-established method; the conventional exercise test (ET), which safeguarded protocols and interpretation, can help to detect diseases, monitor cardiovascular conditions, promote exercise, and reduce the sedentary time for the oldest-old adults [15, 18–22].

Healthy aging identifies a common goal for patients, health professionals, family, and society to optimize FC, with the achievement of five heavily interconnected domains: continuous learning, growth and decision making, mobility, relationship building and maintenance, and contribution for family and society [1]. This study aimed to assess aging, with or without cardiac disease, influences on functional capacity (FC). This assessment is necessary to promote safe, effective, and comfortable exercise for this specific subpopulation. Exercise-based programs for advanced older adults could improve health status, reduce risk factors, and help in managing non-transmissible chronic diseases.

## 3. Functional capacity in advanced older adults: a retrospective study

### 3.1 Methodology

- Sample: obtained from a retrospective medical record review of patients ≥75 years old age (eligible criteria), which had done an exercise test (ET) between 2013 and 2017, performed in a private clinic in the city of Guarapuava, State of Paraná, Brazil. This sample was divided into two groups, according to VO2max (Group A: VO2max <24 ml/kg/min and Group B: ≥24 ml/kg/min). This cutoff number was chosen as a limit of mortality reduction in older adult subpopulation, according to Kokkinos et al. [6].

- Ethical approval: the study was approved by the ethics committee of the Middle West State University of Paraná, (32250020.6.0000.0106, registered in Brazil's Ministry of Health platform).

Procedures:

- Hypothesis: clinical characteristics may be different in varied levels of functional capacity (FC).

- Main objective: to compare and correlate clinical characteristics with FC in advanced elderly.

- Specific objectives: to report sex differences on VO2max, to report other clinical sex differences, and to describe clinical findings in a series of cases in this specific subpopulation.

- Clinical findings definitions: type of recommendation for ET, symptoms prior to ET, personal and family cardiovascular history, traditional RF (hypertension, diabetes, dyslipidemia, smoking, and stress), previously known heart disease, previously known coronary artery disease (CAD), medications including those suspended for ET, and body mass index (BMI). Definitions of hypertension, type 2 diabetes mellitus (DM2), and dyslipidemia were obtained by reporting on anamnesis and use of specific medication. Smoking and stress status were characterized by anamnesis report. CAD was defined by anamnesis and the report of having performed angiocoronariography or coronary tomography with the finding of obstructions, previous revascularization procedures, or acute myocardial infarction confirmed by the executing, the requesting, or compatible changes on the rest electrocardiogram (ECG). The level of activity was defined by self-report, classifying as sedentary or active, based on the time of physical activity per week [12, 18]. Presence of previous heart diseases (ischemic, hypertensive, and valvular heart disease) was recorded by the information of the examinee, ECG alteration compatible with heart disease, or medication for CAD or heart failure. Sedentary or active heart disease patients were also recorded. BMI (weight/height [2]) was obtained from the test report. The following classification was used for BMI: <20: thin, 20–24.9: normal weight, 26–31: overweight; and ≥ 30: obesity [23]. RF were considered alone and grouped by number of RF present in the same individual, being considered for this group: hypertension, DM2, dyslipidemia, smoking, and stress.

- ET and FC methodology: FC was estimated by calculated VO2max obtained on the ET, with methodology according to the III guidelines of the Brazilian Society of Cardiology on exercise testing [21], using adaptable ramp treadmill protocol on an Inbramed ATL treadmill (ANVISA Registration: 10318090009), with data collected and analyzed in the Micromed ErgoPC-13 system (ANVISA Registration: 10307270007) with posterior checkage by the authors. VO2max was calculated using the formula: VO2max = v x (0.073 ± cc / 100) x 1.8, where cc: slope of the treadmill (%) and v: treadmill speed (meters/min) [22]. The other variables were obtained through formulas found in the above-mentioned guideline [21]. All patients were assessed by an ergometry experienced appraiser, which had manually monitored blood pressure with aneroid sphygmomanometer and HR was monitored by ECG. Rest HR was obtained after five min of dorsal decubitus rest. Then, the patient informed data by anamnesis and a clinical exam was done. Stand and hyperpnea ECG registers were taken. Patients initiate effort phase by walking slowly, following an adaptable ramp protocol calculated to reach at least previewed VO2max. Changes in velocity or inclination were done at any time for patient walk comfort. Blood pressure was registered at minutes 0, 2, 5, 8, 11, and 14, as soon as exercise stopped, and in recovery phase, at minutes 1, 2, 3, and 5. ECG registers were taken at minutes 3, 6, 9, 12, and 15 during the exercise phase and minutes 1, 2, 4, and 6 during recovery phase. Exercise phase was interrupted if there were any of the following: exhaustion, limiting symptoms, high-risk ECG findings (ischemia and arrhythmia), or blood pressure limits for normotensive or hypertensive individuals [21].

Group comparison and correlation: groups A and B were compared by sex, BMI, obesity, hypertension, DM2, dyslipidemia, smoking, stress, accumulated RF, activity level, presence of heart disease, presence of known CAD, indication for ET, symptoms till the date of ET, duration of exertion phase, distance covered, symptoms to ET, reasons for interruption of ET, New York Heart Association classification, systolic blood pressure (SBP) in all phases, diastolic blood pressure in all phases, SBP variation (delta), delta SPB/MET, pressure responses to ET, rest HR, HR of the peak of exertion, HR in the sixth minute of recovery, HR reserve, recovery of HR, sum of reserves, gradient of reserves, resting ECG, ECG during exercise phase, ECG in recovery phase, and the presence of arrhythmias, Duke score, and final report. Comparations between some of these factors and correlations between the most highlighted factors were also performed.

- Statistical analysis: for the comparison of continuous values, a two-tailed Student's t-test was used, and, for categorical variables, chi-square test ($chi^2$) with Yates' correction was performed. Spearman and Pearson's correlation tests were used to associate factors with VO2max and factors with each other. Multivariate regression analysis was performed to evaluate if any factor would have the ability to predict VO2max. The regression analysis was preceded by assessment of variable linearity on the linear graphic, normality by Kolmogorov–Smirnov test, independence by two-sample means t-statistics test, and homoscedasticity with Levène's test. If heteroscedasticity was detected, white test and Breusch-Pagan test were performed for residual analysis. The statistical tests were performed by SPSS Statistics-IBM (2018) software, except the heteroscedasticity tests, which were done by Gretl 2021b (2021) software. Significant results were considered with $p \leq 0.05$. Results related to the same problem, such as the characteristics derived from HR and BP; formulas in which one factor is part of the estimation of another, such as cardiac output and blood pressure, were considered as possible confounders.

## 3.2 Results

We observed that women were in majority in this study and had more reported dyslipidemia, reported cumulative risk factors (RF) and reported sedentary behavior associated with cardiopathy and rest electrocardiogram (ECG) changes than men. There was trend for more obesity in women, but Yates' correction did not confirm chi2 result. Other baseline findings, such as age, body mass index (BMI), hypertension, diabetes mellitus, smoking, stress, previous coronary artery disease (CAD) recommendations for exercise test (ET), symptoms present before ET, and foreseen and obtained maximal oxygen uptake (VO2máx), did not differ between sexes.

In comparative analysis, Among the categorical variables, there was a difference in the comparison in ET indication, blood pressure responses, and obesity, when comparing A group with B group. ECG changes tended to be more frequent in A group, but chi2 result was not confirmed by Yates' correction. Categorical variables such as activity level, symptoms before ET, cumulative RF, hypertension, diabetes mellitus, dyslipidemia, smoking, and stress were not different in both groups. The continuous variables analysis showed a difference between the groups for BMI and heart rate (HR) reserve. There were no differences in age, blood pressure measures, and other HR measures (**Table 1**).

Rest HR was correlated with BMI with weak intensity, but there was no correlation with peak HR and HR Reserve (**Figure 1**).

Pre-regression analysis was done as reported in **Table 2**., with obtained assumptions: dependent and independent values were continuous, linearity on correlation dispersion graphics, independence with independent samples confidence interval, and normality by the Kolmogorov–Smirnov's test. Variance homogeneity could not be assumed after applying the Levène's test. White and Breusch-Pagan's tests for heterogenicity of variances did not reject homoscedasticity, and regression was proceeded.

| | Category | A (n = 29) | B (n = 57) | p |
|---|---|---|---|---|
| Age (years) | — | 79.3 ± 3.4 | 78.1 ± 3.5 | 0.114 (t) |
| ET indication | Symptoms assessment | 12(41.4) | 13(22.8) | 0.034 (chi$^2$) |
| | Known CAD | 2(6.9) | 11(19.3) | |
| | Risk factors | 13(44.8) | 31(54.4) | |
| | Arrhythmias | 2(6.9) | 2(3.5) | |
| ECG | Normal | 8(27.6) | 6(10.5) | 0.042 (chi$^2$, Yates:0.089) |
| | Discrete changes | 18(6.7) | 43(75.4) | |
| | Significant changes | 3(11.3) | 8 (14.1) | |
| Rest SBP | Depressed | 1(3.5) | 5(8.7) | 0.008 (chi$^2$) |
| | Exacerbated | 15(51.7) | 11(19.3) | |
| | Normal | 13(44.8) | 41(72.0) | |
| Rest DBP | Exacerbated | 2(6.9) | 0 | 0.047 (chi$^2$) |
| | Normal | 27(93.1) | 57(100) | |
| BMI (kg/m$^2$) | — | 28.4 ± 4.1 | 26.7 ± 3.4 | 0.045 (t) |
| Obesity (BMI ≥ 30) | — | 12(41.3) | 10 (17.5) | 0.017 (chi$^2$) |
| HR reserve (bpm) | — | 49 ± 17 | 56 ± 14 | 0.043 (t) |

*Continuous variables are expressed in means. ET: Exercise test, ECG: electrocardiogram, SBP: systolic blood pressure, DBP: diastolic blood pressure, CAD: coronary artery disease, A: A group, VO2max < 24 mg/kg/min, B: B group, VO2max ≥ 24 ml/kg/min, BMI: body mass index, SBP: systolic blood pressure, Delta SBP: peak SBP – rest SBP, HR reserve: peak heart rate – rest heart rate, A: A group (VO2max < 24 mg/kg/min), B: B group (VO2max ≥ 24 mg/kg/min), t = Student's t-test, Chi$^2$: chi-square test (Source: authors).*

**Table 1.**
*Main comparisons between VO2max groups.*

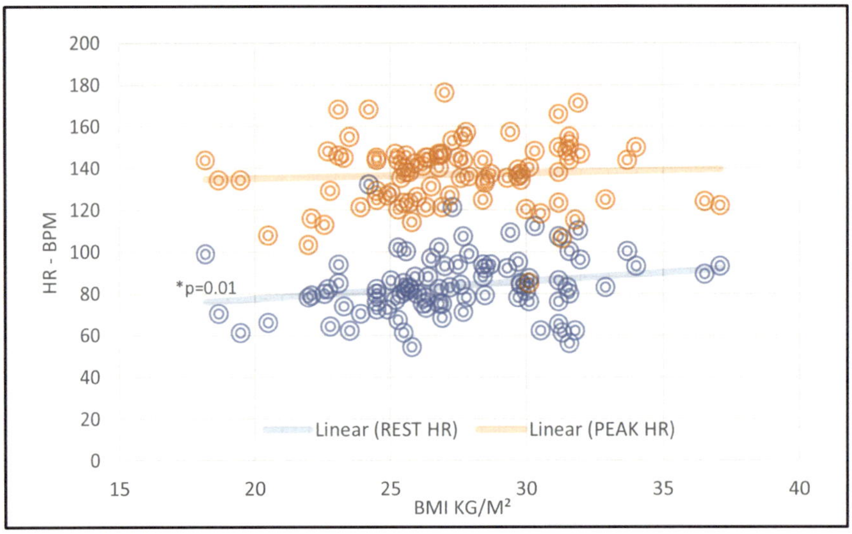


**Figure 1.**
*Correlation between HR and BMI. HR: Heart rate, BMI: Body mass index (weight/height$^2$), data presented in averages, linear correlation *p = 0.01, Spearman's rho = 0.272. (source: Authors).*

| Analysis | Test | Result | Interpretation |
|---|---|---|---|
| Continuous variables | — | three continuous variables: VO2max, rest HR, and BMI | Assumed |
| Linearity | Graphic analysis | Linear dispersion | Assumed |
| Independence | Independent Samples Confidence Interval | VO2max/BMI: CI (95%) = 0.9 ± 1.6<br>VO2max/Rest HR: CI (95%) = 810.6 ± 31.1<br>Rest HR/BMI: CI (95%) = 809.7 ± 31.1 | Assumed |
| Normality | Kolmogorov–Smirnov | VO2max: K-S = 0.846 p = 0.542<br>BMI: K-S = 0.056 p = 0.938<br>Rest HR: K-S = 0.797, p = 0.618 | Assumed |
| Homoscedasticity | Levène | VO2max/IMC: f = 13.192, p˂0.01<br>VO2max/Rest HR: f = 35.678 p < 0.01<br>Rest HR/BMI: f = 65.120 p < 0.01 | Not assumed |
| Heteroscedasticity | White<br>Breusch-Pagan | TR^2 = 4.4412, p = 0.488<br>LM = 6.5943 p = 0.037 | Not rejected |

*VO2max: maximal oxygen uptake. HR: heart rate, BMI: body mass index, CI: confidence interval, K-S: Kolmogorov–Smirnov index, f ratio: Levène index, TR^2: White index, LM: Breusch-Pagan index (Source: authors).*

**Table 2.**
*Pre-regression analysis.*

Linear regression analysis observed a linear correlation between rest HR, VO2max, and BMI, with following Pearson's test results (BMI and VO2max, $r(84) = -0.214$, $p = 0.05$; HR and VO2max, $r(84) = 0.211$, $p = 0.05$; and HR and BMI, $r(84) = 0.208$, $p = 0.05$). Although not all assumptions were reached, multivariate regression returned a prediction formula, in which the rest of HR predicts VO2max at different BMI levels (**Figure 2**).

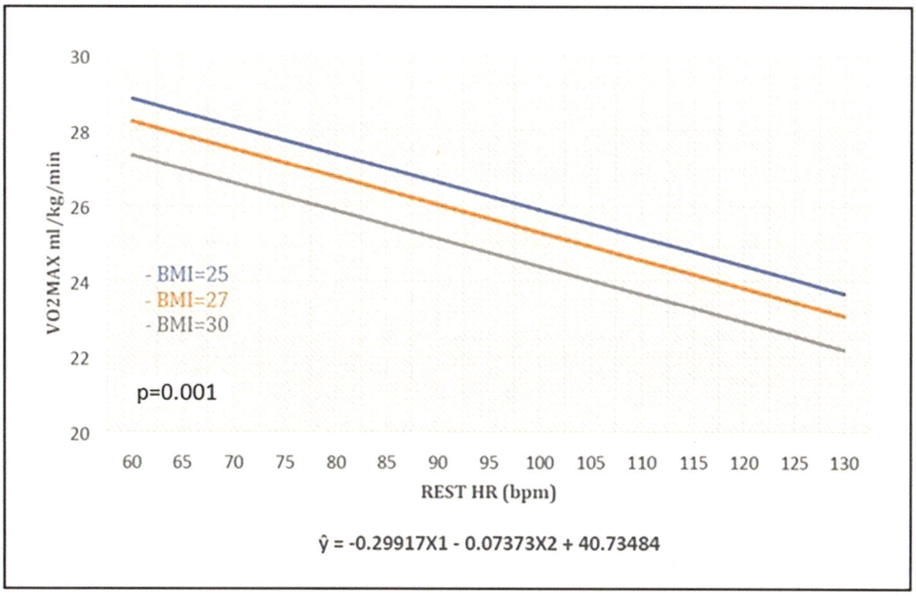


**Figure 2.**
*Multivariate regression equation applied to three BMI value, rest HR, and BMI. Data presented in linear value, bivariate regression analysis p = 0.001. (Source: authors).*

### 3.3 Discussion

This case series (n = 86) has an average age of 78.5 years, which is superior to life expectancy in Brazil (76 years) [2]. Risk factors (RF) incidence in oldest-old adults, when compared with Vivacqua et al. [24], is similar for sedentary behavior (75.5% x 77%); but different for hypertension (83.7% x 21%), dyslipidemia (53.5% x 22%), smoking (9.3% x 3%), and diabetes mellitus (16.3% x 6%). In the Vacanti, Sespedes, and Sarpi [25] series, 50% there were hypertensive, 36% had dyslipidemia, and 14% were diabetics. Sedentary behavior is linked to more than 36 pathological situations [12]. This survey observed 75.6% self-declared sedentary, but this data may be underestimated, as it is obtained by self-report [23]. Sedentary behavior was more frequently declared by patients with cardiac disease, and it is concerning because exercise is a therapeutic resource for almost all types of cardiac diseases [26]. This sample showed 17.4% of known coronary artery disease (CAD) and 14% of ischemia signs on exercise test (ET). Women declared more dyslipidemia, cumulative RF, with a trend for obesity. Hormonal protection seems to disappear a few years after menopause and RF prevalence rises in females [27]. Data about sedentary behavior, BMI, and RF are aligned with epidemiological studies, which report low adherence of older adults to health goals composed by RF control, dietary changes, and physical activity [28]. RF and VO2max have been reported as significant markers of cardiovascular disease and mortality in this age group [18].

Symptoms before ET were reported by 46.5%, more than observed in the Vacanti, Sespedes, and Sarpi [25] study, which found 35% of symptomatic examinees. Recommendations for ET were RF assessment (51.2%), symptoms assessment (29,1%) e CAD follow up (15.1%). Vivacqua et al. [24], in a male-predominant and in hospital laboratory sample, found these recommendations: exercise capacity assessment (61%), therapeutic assessment (22%), post-myocardial infarction

(17%), post-myocardial revascularization (10%), post-angioplasty (5%), and chest pain assessment (1%). Adaptable ramp protocol [20] for treadmill ET was applied in all patients, with 97.7% of cases reaching exhaustion at the end of exercise phase. Another study in the same age group, but with adaptable Bruce protocol, average length of exercise phase was 6.8 ± 2 minutes [25], different from this sample with an average length of 10.3 ± 2,4 minutes. This exercise phase lenght average is recomended by Brazilian guidelines on ET ramp protocol [21]. During ET, few cases presented symptoms, such as angina (1.2%) and dyspnea (3.5%). Only two cases presented exercise-limiting symptoms. These data are like other studies in oldest-old adults [20, 22, 27] and suggest ET is a safe procedure in this subpopulation.

The VO2max average (26.4 ± 6.20) obtained was superior to previewed for men (26.9 x 22.4 ml/kg/min) and women (25.9 x 14.7 ml/kg/min). Vivacqua et al. [24] observed lower values: 20.6 ml/kg/min for men and 19.6 ml/kg/min for women and Vacanti, Sespedes, and Sarpi [25] found average of 23.1 ml/kg/min. When compared to averages of this study, it should be reasonable to think about a functional increase of oldest-old adults in the last decades, on the other hand, studies with in-hospital samples may have included more severe cases. Eriksen et al. [29] evaluated 16,025 individuals, 1077 over 70 years old age, with cycle ET, and found correlation between active time and sedentary time with mortality. They also found average VO2max values closer to the observed in the present study: 29.7 ml/kg/min (men) and 24.1 ml/kg/min (women). Ferrari and Goelzer [20], with an octogenary sample submitted to treadmill ET, found a VO2max range of 20.8–22.7 ml/kg/min (men) and 16.5–19.2 ml/kg/min (women). If considered only individuals ≥80 years, this study found higher averages: 24.6 ml/kg/min (men) e 24.4 ml/kg/min (women). Using cardiopulmonary stress test (CST), Almeida et al. [17] evaluated 103 individuals with more than 70 years old, without cardiac disease, and found average values of 22.06 ± 4.7 ml/kg/min (men) and 17.41 ± 3.7 ml/kg/min (women) in the 70–79 group; and 19.20 ± 3.4 ml/kg/min (men) e 16.56 ± 2.9 ml/kg/min (women) for the ≥80 years old group. The VO2max averages presented here are higher, and this could be explained by method differences, reported by Lima et al. [30], who found that calculated VO2max is overestimated by 15–38% when compared to measured VO2max in a CST. Kokkinos et al. [31], assessing 5314 old men with treadmill ET, observed inverse correlation between mortality and exercise capacity with a VO2max neutral point of 17.5 ml/kg/min. Recently, the same group found VO2max thresholds for 10-year mortality by age groups, the over 70 years old group should have 24% of mortality reduction in the VO2max range 21–28 ml/kg/min [6]. Same findings were observed by Mandsager et al. [32] in a sample of 122,007 older adults. In the same way, Korpelainen et al. [33], with 3,033 older adults on treadmill ET, observed that FC was the strongest indicator of cardiovascular and general mortality.

Rest HR average was 83.7 bpm, the exercise peak was 137 bpm, and HR reserve was 53.3b pm, like Vacanti, Sespedes and Sarpi [25], which found 82.6 bpm at rest, 134.2 bpm at exercise peak, and a HR reserve of 51.6 bpm. In the present study, 16.3% had normal ECG, 70.9% had discrete changes, and 12.8% had significant changes. Women's rest ECG had more changes than men's rest ECG. Only 7.0% of all samples presented significant ST changes during ET, contrasting with Vivacqua et al. [24] in-hospital samples, which found significant ST changes in 22%.

Comparison of two VO2max groups showed some significant differences. Recommendations for ET to assess symptoms, lower HR reserve, abnormal blood pressure response, and higher BMI were more frequent in A group, with lower VO2max (**Table 1**). Fernandes-silva et al. [34], in a populational study, found a direct and independent correlation between BMI and arterial stiffness in older adults, which is a marker of future cardiac disease. A Chinese study with oldest-old adults showed that low weight was associated with higher mortality, and overweight was associated with lower mortality rate than normal weight [35]. Park et al. [36] associated older adults' weight maintenance with low mortality rate; great loss of weight was associated with higher mortality and weight gain was associated with mild elevation of mortality. Abnormal blood pressure responses, systolic and diastolic, were higher in the A group (**Table 1**), this abnormal response has been linked to future hypertension, atherosclerosis, cognitive disorders, and mortality [30].

A weak correlation between BMI and rest HR was observed, but not with peak HR or HR reserve (**Figure 1**). Rest HR and obesity have been associated with development of cardiac disease [37] and atrial fibrillation, as well as mortality, in older adults [38, 39].

Multivariate regression showed interrelation between BMI, rest HR, and VO2max indicating that for higher rest HR and higher BMI, lower levels of VO2max are expected. These results, however, should be seen with caution, because of some statistical limitations, such as the non-homogeneity of variance in these sample values. Since the White and Breusch-Pagan tests had not rejected homoscedasticity (**Table 2**), the regression is presented (**Figure 2**) but considered unable to purpose a prediction model. Forman et al. [20] suggest that exercise capacity remains a target for therapeutic management in the elderly, emphasizing hemodynamic strategies, such as rest HR and metabolic approach, including BMI, with simple approaches, such as dietary intervention and physical activity.

This study has many limitations: VO2max was calculated, not measured, so values may be overestimated. The ex-post-fact context is limiting because clinical characteristics were self-related and there was no possibility to apply validated questionnaires. Sample size may not allow to demonstrate more significant results, and there is possible bias in regression results caused by sample heteroscedasticity. In this study, it was impossible to establish prediction of VO2max based on resting heart rate or body mass index, but it could be an idea for future research. Despite limitations, this study suggests a practical implication: this subpopulation can benefit from a pre-participation assessment of clinical and functional capacity features, followed by exercise prescription, another one is that it could support the development of strategies for active aging programs [1, 40] and healthcare delivery to oldest-old adults [19, 24].

## 4. Promoting physical activity for advanced older adults

The practice of health-promoting and therapeutic physical activity, with minimal risks, is also a factor in the development of autonomy, self-esteem, and comprehensiveness of care. Such a measure can aid in sociability when adopted in therapeutic groups [41], helps in psychomotricity [42], improves cognitive performance [43], promotes the control of various cardiovascular risk factors [44], reduces the cancer risk [45], and favors lower risk of falls and fractures [46]. There is also evidence that regular physical activity can attenuate the effects of aging on the cardiovascular system [47, 48]. Therefore, it is necessary to approach interdisciplinary and create simple and reproducible and easy-expanding programs to promote physical activity for this subpopulation. These programs should consider the natural aging process and the fact that these people reach advanced ages bringing with them diseases, sequelae, cultural and environmental issues, preferences, and social conditions obtained throughout a lifetime. Exercise in the elderly is considered as promoter of quality of life with improvement of physical, social, and emotional aspects; mortality reduction, especially cardiovascular mortality; reducing the risk of cancer; and prevention of falls. There is, therefore, the need for reception, equity, attention to cultural aspects, and care for psychosocial situations, aiming for adherence and effectiveness [40].

Exercises of the most varied modalities can bring benefit to the health of the elderly, such as aerobic, resisted, or combined [48]. Smolarek et al. [49], observed that, in old women trained for 12 weeks with strength exercises, there was an improvement in both the strength of the limbs and the cognition indexes. It is possible to improve functional capacity with training even in the elderly; a systematic review showed that most studies found favorable results in physical capacity and psychological aspects in the elderly undergoing various forms of structured training [50].

Health system structure, and society in general, should be aware of the growing demands of this population on physical activity and requires clinical and complementary evaluation, where the ET is included as a tool capable of giving prognostic information, functional data, and motivation for the mobilization of the elderly because there is a high prevalence of sedentary lifestyle among the elderly, which remains unchanged for decades [28]. Exercise should be focused on the improvement of FC [1]. Managers and health professionals who work with the elderly cannot be satisfied with only accepting the nonadherence to exercise but should look for the causes of nonaccess and break these barriers [40].

## 5. Resistance training in older adults

The more obvious benefit of resistance training for advanced older adults is the prevention of muscular decline, which is achieved by gene and protein expression in muscle cells, with individual heterogeneity, delivering shift in the muscle fibers, muscle mass gain, force, power, mobility, and balance improvement [51]. Studies with resistance training programs (RTP) for older adults have been published in last three decades, and main results were compiled in a meta-analysis by Liu and Latham [52], with 121 studies and 6700 patients. They observed a favorable result for resistance exercise in physical function improvement in older adults. RTP is considered safe and is associated with retarding aging of muscle mass, muscle strength improvement, and reducing chronic inflammation [53]. RTP is recommended for healthy and frail individuals, with limits and technics personalization [51]. These results, achieved by neuromuscular and neuroendocrine adaptations, can help patients to improve mobility, functional capacity, performance in activities of daily living, and preserve the independence, with a dose–response effectivity relationship [54, 55]. RTP have been associated to better quality of life [56], reducing frailty symptoms [57], retarding cognitive decline [58], preventing sarcopenia and falls [59], and lowering risks of cardiovascular disease and all-cause mortality [60], with significant impact of BMI on these two major events [61]. The use of RTP can even reduce social and geographic barriers that affect elderly [62]. Cardiovascular benefits have been described, as reducing arterial stiffness [63] and blood pressure [64]. RTP can also help to improve FC in older adults, a meta-analysis with 22 studies reported that within 24-week programs, there was a 2.57 ml/kg/min mean gain in VO2max, assessed by ET [65]. In heart failure patients, RTP achieved an improvement of muscle strength, quality of life, and FC [66]. There is a recent report of FC gain in older women survivors of breast cancer, which is an important aim because quality of life and insulin resistance are associated with recidivism [67]. Even advanced pulmonary cancer patients have been trained with RTP with favorable results in quality of life and physical function [68, 69]. A systematic review observed quality of life and survival improvements in cancer survivors with regular exercise practice, most of studies were on RTP programs [70]. In order to assist the elderly in achieving FC improvements, therefore, an interdisciplinary approach, involving various health professionals, a support team, and health managers could be very helpful [71].

## 6. Conclusions

This study allowed us to conclude that advanced older adults, compared by functional capacity (VO2max cutoff = 24 mg/kg/min), had significant differences in important factors: heart rate reserve, body mass index, recommendation to assess symptoms, and abnormal blood pressure response. We also found a correlation between resting heart rate and body mass index, and both to functional capacity. Since these variables have been associated with higher risks of disease and mortality in older adults in a great number of studies. As a practical implication, we reinforce that oldest-old adults can benefit from a pre-participation assessment of clinical and functional capacity features, followed by exercise prescription to get the final objective of active aging. These findings can also support exercise programs, resistance training included, which are important tools to achieve this objective.

## Author notes

Review and research developed under the Interdisciplinary Post Graduate Program in Community Development, Middle West State University of Paraná, for master's degree obtaining, in Guarapuava, Paraná, Brazil.

## Author details

Abrão José Melhem Junior[1*], Miguel Morita Fernandes-Silva[2]
and David Livingstone Alves Figueiredo[1]

1 Medicine Department, Middle West State University of Paraná, UNICENTRO, Brazil

2 Internal Medicine Department, Federal University of Paraná, UFPR, Brazil

*Address all correspondence to: amelhem@unicentro.br

## References

[1] World Health Organization - WHO. World report on ageing and health. World Health Organization (WHO/OMS). 2015. Available from: https://www.who.int/ageing/publications/world-report-2015/en/ [Accessed 2019 July 30]

[2] Brasil. Instituto Brasileiro de Geografia e Estatística - IBGE. Projeção populacional. 2019. Available from: https://www.ibge.gov.br/apps/populacao/projecao/ [Accessed 2019 July 25]

[3] Lee IM, Shiroma EJ, Kamasa M, Basset DR, Matthews CE, Buring JE, et al. Association of step volume and intensity with all-cause mortality in older women. Journal of the American Medical Association. 2019;**179**(8):1105-1113

[4] Khan H, Nabil J, Rauramaa R, Sudhir K, Kai S, Laukkanen JA, et al. Cardiorespiratory fitness and non-fatal cardiovascular events: A population-based follow-up study. American Heart Journal. 2017;**184**:55-61

[5] Bourgeois FT, Orenstein L, Ballakur S, Mandl KD, Ioannidis JP. Exclusion of elderly persons in randomized clinical trials of drugs for ischemic heart disease. Journal of the American Geriatrics Society. 2017;**65**(11):2354-2361

[6] Kokkinos P, Faselis C, Myers J, Sui X, Zhang J, Blair S. Age-specific exercise capacity threshold for mortality risk assessment in male veterans. Circulation. 2014;**130**(8):653-658

[7] Faselis C, Kokkinos P, Tsimploulis A, Pittaras A, Myers J, Lavie CJ, et al. Exercise capacity and all-cause mortality in male veterans with hypertension aged ≥70 years. Hypertension. 2014;**64**(1):30-35

[8] Monteverde M, Noronha K, Palloni A, Novak AB. Obesity and excess mortality among the elderly in the United States and Mexico. Demography. 2010;**47**(1):79-96

[9] Tamakoshi A, Yatsuya H, Lin Y, Tamakoshi K, Kondo T, Suzuki S, et al. BMI and all-cause mortality among Japanese older adults: Findings from the Japan collaborative cohort study. Obesity. 2009;**18**(2):362-369

[10] Stessman J, Jacobs JM, Ein-Mor E, Bursztyn M. Normal body mass index rather than obesity predicts greater mortality in elderly people: The Jerusalem longitudinal study. Journal of the American Geriatrics Society. 2009;**57**(12):2232-2238

[11] Wajngaarten M, Sanches PCR. Processo natural do envelhecimento cardiovascular. In: In: BORGES, Jairo Lins., editor. Manual de Cardiogeraitria. 4th ed. São Paulo: Leitura Médica; 2018. pp. 17-25

[12] Booth FW, Roberts CK, Thyfault JP, Ruegsegger GN, Toedebusch RG. Role of inactivity in chronic diseases: Evolutionary insight and pathophysiological mechanisms. Physiological Reviews. 2017;**97**(4):1351-1402

[13] Li CM, Chang CI, Wen-Ruey Y, Yang W, Hsub CC, Chen CY. Enhancing elderly health examination effectiveness by adding physical function evaluations and interventions. Archives of Gerontology and Geriatrics. 2017;**70**:38-43

[14] Rodrigues R, Silva C, Loureiro L, Silva S, Crespo S, Azeredo Z. The oldest old: Multidimensional functional assessment. Revista de Enfermagem. 2015;**5**:65-74

[15] Borges JL. Investigação de doença coronária no idoso. In: Borges JL, editor. Manual de Cardiogeriatria. 4th ed. São Paulo: Leitura Médica; 2018. pp. 27-44

[16] Kim BJ, Youngju K, Oh J, Jang J, Kang SK. Characteristics and safety of cardiopulmonary exercise testing in elderly patients with cardiovascular diseases in Korea. Yonsei Medical Journal. 2019;**60**(6):547-550

[17] Almeida AE, Santander IR, Campos MI, Arévalo JR, Nascimento JA, Ritt LE. Classification system for cardiorespiratory fitness based on a sample of the Brazilian population. International Journal of Cardiovascular Sciences. 2019:343-354

[18] Ross R, Blair SN, Arena R, Church TS, Després JP, Franklin BA, et al. Importance of assessing cardiorespiratory fitness in clinical practice: A case for fitness as a clinical vital sign. Circulation. 2016;**134**(24):653-699

[19] Forman DE, Arena R, Boxer R, Dolansky MA, Eng JJ, Fleg JL, et al. Prioritizing functional capacity as a principal end point for therapies oriented to older adults with cardiovascular disease: A scientific statement for healthcare professionals from the American Heart Association. Circulation. 2017;**135**(16):894-918

[20] Ferrari E, Goelzer LS. Protocolo em Rampa para octogenários modificado. Revista do Derc. 2017;**23**(3):74-76

[21] Meneghelo RS, Araújo CG, Stein R, Mastrocolla LE, Albuquerque PF, Serra SM et al./Sociedade Brasileira de Cardiologia. III Diretrizes da Sociedade Brasileira de Cardiologia sobre teste ergométrico. Arquivos Brasileiros de Cardiologia 2010;95(5, supl.1): 1-26.

[22] Balke B, Ware RW. The Present Status of Physical Fitness in the Air Force. Texas: School of Aviation Medicine. Randolph Air Force Base; 1959

[23] Lipschitz DA. Screening for nutritional status in the elderly. Primary Care. 1994;**21**(1):55-67

[24] Vivacqua R, Serra S, Macaciel R, Miranda M, Bueno N, Campos A. Teste ergométrico em idosos. Parâmetros Clínicos, Metabólicos, Hemodinâmicos e Eletrocardiográficos. Arquivos Brasileiros de Cardiologia. 1997;**68**(1):9-12

[25] Vacanti LJ, Sespedes LB, Sarpi MO. O teste ergométrico é útil, seguro e eficaz, mesmo em indivíduos muito idosos, com 75 anos ou mais. Arquivos Brasileiros de Cardiologia. 2004;**82**(2):147-150

[26] Korose S, Iwasaka J, Tsutsumi H, Yamanaka Y, Shinno H, Fukushima Y, et al. Effect of exercise-based cardiac rehabilitation on non-culprit mild coronary plaques in the culprit coronary artery of patients with acute coronary syndrome. Heart and Vessels. 2015;**31**(6):846-854

[27] Gravina CF, Rosa RF, Franken RA, Freitas EV, Liberman A, et al. II Diretrizes Brasileiras em Cardiogeriatria. Arquivos Brasileiros de Cardiologia. 2010;**95**(3 supl.2):1-112

[28] Mozaffarian D, Benjamin EJ, Go AS, Arnett DK, Blaha MJ, Cushman M, et al. Heart disease and stroke statistics—2015 update. Circulation. 27 Jan 2015;**131**(4):e29-322

[29] Eriksen L, Grønbæk M, Helge JW, Tolstrup JS. Cardiorespiratory fitness in 16 025 adults aged 18-91 years and associations with physical activity and sitting time. Scandinavian Journal of Medicine & Science in Sports. 2015;**26**(12):1435-1443

[30] Lima RM, Bottaro M, Rauber SB, Moreira SR, Carregaro RL, Barros JF, et al.

Exaggerated blood pressure response during the exercise treadmill test as a risk factor for hypertension. Brazilian Journal of Medical and Biological Research. 2013;**46**(4):338-347

[31] Kokkinos P, Myers J, Faselis C, Panagiotakos DB, Doumas M, Pittaras A, et al. Exercise capacity and mortality in older men. Circulation. 2010;**122**(8):790-797

[32] Mandsager K, Harb S, Cremer P, Phelan D, Nissen SE, Jaber W. Association of cardiorespiratory fitness with long-term mortality among adults undergoing exercise treadmill testing. JAMA Network Open. 2018;**1**(6):1-12

[33] Korpelainen R, Lämsä J, Kaikkonen KM, Korpelainen J, Laukkanen J, Palatsiet I, et al. Exercise capacity and mortality – A follow-up study of 3033 subjects referred to clinical exercise testing. Annals of Medicine. 2016;**48**(5):359-366

[34] Fernandes-Silva MM, Shah AM, Claggett B, Cheng S, Tanaka H, Silvestre IM, et al. Adiposity, body composition and ventricular-arterial stiffness in the elderly: The atherosclerosis risk in communities study. European Journal of Heart Failure. 2018;**20**(8):1191-1201

[35] Wang J, Taylor AW, Zhang T, Appleton S, Shi Z. Association between body mass index and all-cause mortality among oldest old Chinese. The Journal of Nutrition, Health & Aging. 2017;**22**(2):262-268

[36] Park SY, Wilkens LR, Maskarinec G, Haiman CA, Kolonel LN, Marchand LL, et al. Weight change in older adults and mortality: The multiethnic cohort study: The multiethnic cohort study. International Journal of Obesity. 2017;**42**(2):205-212

[37] Izeli NL, Santos AJ, Crescêncio JC, Gonçalves AC, Papa V, Marques F, et al. Aerobic training after myocardial infarction: Remodeling evaluated by cardiac magnetic resonance. Arquivos Brasileiros de Cardiologia. 2016;**106**(4):311-318

[38] Aladin AI, Rifai MA, Rasool SH, Keteyian SJ, Brawner CA, Blumenthal RS, et al. Relation of resting heart rate to incident atrial fibrillation (from the Henry ford hospital exercise testing project). The American Journal of Cardiology. 2017;**119**(2):262-267

[39] Foy AJ, Mandrola J, Liu G, Naccarelli GV. Relation of obesity to new-onset atrial fibrillation and atrial flutter in adults. The American Journal of Cardiology. 2018;**121**(9):1072-1075

[40] Mora JC, Valencia WM. Exercise and older adults. Clinics in Geriatric Medicine. 2018;**34**(1):145-162

[41] Meurer ST, Benedetti TRB, Mazo GZ. Aspectos da autoimagem e autoestima de idosos ativos. Motriz. 2009;**15**(4):788-796

[42] Rubira APFA et al. Efeito de exercícios psicomotores no equilíbrio de idosos. Conscientiae Saúde. 2014;**13**(1):54-61

[43] Merege-filho CAA et al. Influência do exercício físico na cognição: uma atualização sobre mecanismos fisiológicos. Revista Brasileira de Medicina do Esporte. 2014;**20**(3):237-241

[44] Gravina CF et al. 2ª Diretriz de Cardiogeriatria. da Sociedade Brasileira de Cardiologia. Arquivos Brasileiros de Cardiologia. 2010;**95**(3):s2

[45] Moore SC et al. Association of Leisure-Time physical activity with risk of 26 types of cancer in 1.44 million adults. JAMA Internal Medicine. 2016;**176**(6):816

[46] Cunha P, Pinheiro LC. O papel do exercício físico na prevenção das quedas nos idosos: uma revisão baseada na evidência. Revista Portuguesa de Medicina Geral e Familiar. 2016;**32**:96-100

[47] Kwak HB. Aging, exercise, and extracellular matrix in the heart. Journal of Exercise Rehabilitation. 2013;**9**(3):338-347

[48] Garber CE, Blissmer B, Deschenes MR, Franklin BA, Lamonte MJ, Lee IM, et al. Quantity and quality of exercise for developing and maintaining cardiorespiratory, musculoskeletal, and neuromotor fitness in apparently healthy adults. Medicine & Science in Sports & Exercise. 2011;**43**(7):1334-1359

[49] Smolarek AC, Ferreira LHB, Schoenfeld B, Cordeiro GR, Alessi A, Laat EF, et al. Cognitive performance changes after a 12-week strength training program in overweight older women. Journal of Exercise Physiology Online. 2019;**22**(5):1-9

[50] Souza WC, Mascarenhas LPG, Grzelczak MT, Tajes Junior D, Brasilino FF, Lima VA. Exercício físico na promoção da saúde na terceira idade. Saúde & Meio Ambiente: Revista Interdisciplinar. 2015;**4**(1):55-65

[51] Lavin KM, Roberts BM, Fry CS, Moro T, Rasmussen BB, Bamman MM. The importance of resistance exercise training to combat neuromuscular aging. Physiology (Bethesda, Md.). 2019;**34**(2):112-122

[52] Liu CJ, Latham NK. Progressive resistance strength training for improving physical function in older adults. Cochrane Database of Systematic Reviews. 8 Jul 2009;**2009**(3):CD002759. DOI: 10.1002/14651858.CD002759.pub2. PMID: 19588334; PMCID: PMC4324332

[53] Sardeli AV, Tomeleri CM, Cyrino ES, et al. Effect of resistance training on inflammatory markers of older adults: A meta-analysis. Experimental Gerontology. 2018;**111**:188-196

[54] Fragala MS, Cadore EL, Dorgo S, Izquierdo M, Kraemer WJ, Peterson MD, et al. Resistance training for older adults: Position statement from the national strength and conditioning association. Journal of Strength and Conditioning Research. 2019;**33**(8):2019-2052

[55] Steib S, Schoene D, Pfeifer K. Dose–response relationship of resistance training in older adults: A meta-analysis. Medicine and Science in Sports and Exercise. 2010;**42**(5):902-914

[56] Syed-Abdul M, McClellan C, Parks E, Ball S. Effects of a resistance training community programme in older adults. Ageing and Society. 2022;**42**(8):1863-1878

[57] Nagai K, Myamato T, Okamae A, et al. Physical activity combined with resistance training reduces symptoms of frailty in older adults: A randomized controlled trial. Archives of Gerontology and Geriatrics. 2018;**76**:41-47

[58] Li Z, Peng X, Xiang W, et al. The effect of resistance training on cognitive function in the older adults: A systematic review of randomized clinical trials. Aging Clinical and Experimental Research. 2018;**30**:1259-1273

[59] Rodrigues F, Domingos C, Monteiro D, Morouço P. A review on aging, sarcopenia, falls, and resistance training in community-dwelling older adults. International Journal of Environmental Research and Public Health. 2022;**19**(2):874

[60] Liu Y, Lee DC, Li Y, et al. Associations of resistance exercise with cardiovascular disease morbidity and

mortality. Medicine and Science in Sports and Exercise. 2019;**51**(3):499-508

[61] Saeidifard F, Medina-Inojosa JR, West CP, et al. The association of resistance training with mortality: A systematic review and meta-analysis. European Journal of Preventive Cardiology. 2019;**26**(15):1647-1665

[62] Baker BS, Miller K, Weitzel KJ, Duren DL, Gammon R, Mills-Gray S, et al. Resistance training reduces age- and geography-related physical function discrepancies in older adults. Gerontology Geriatric Medicine. 2021;**5**(7):233

[63] Shiotsu Y, Watanabe Y, Tujii S, Yanagita M. Effect of exercise order of combined aerobic and resistance training on arterial stiffness in older men. Experimental Gerontology. 2018;**111**:27-34

[64] Herrod PJJ, Doleman B, Blackwell JEM, O'Boyle F, Williams JP, Lund JN, et al. Exercise and other nonpharmacological strategies to reduce blood pressure in older adults: A systematic review and meta-analysis. Journal of the American Society of Hypertension. 2018;**12**(4):248-267

[65] Smart TFF, Doleman B, Hatt J, Paul M, Toft S, Lund JN, et al. The role of resistance exercise training for improving cardiorespiratory fitness in healthy older adults: A systematic review and meta-analysis. Age and Ageing. 2022;**51**(6):afac143

[66] Giuliano C, Karahalios A, Neil C, Allen J, Levinger I. The effects of resistance training on muscle strength, quality of life and aerobic capacity in patients with chronic heart failure - a meta-analysis. International Journal of Cardiology. 2017;**227**:413-423

[67] Winters-Stone KM, Torgrimson-Ojerio B, Dieckmann NF, Stoyles S, Mitri Z, Luoh SW. A randomized-controlled trial comparing supervised aerobic training to resistance training followed by unsupervised exercise on physical functioning in older breast cancer survivors. Journal of Geriatric Oncology. 2022;**13**(2):152-160

[68] Tatematsu N, Naito T, Okayama T, et al. Development of home-based resistance training for older patients with advanced cancer: The exercise component of the nutrition and exercise treatment for advanced cancer program. Journal of Geriatric Oncology. 2021;**12**(6):952-955

[69] Mikkelsen MK, Lund CM, Vinther A, et al. Effects of a 12-week multimodal exercise intervention among older patients with advanced Cancer: Results from a randomized controlled trial. The Oncologist. 2022;**27**(1):67-78

[70] Melhem AJJ, Cordeiro GR, Mascarenhas LPG, Figueiredo DLA. Impacto da atividade física na qualidade de vida e sobrevida de idosos com câncer: uma revisão sistemática. Estudos Interdisciplinares Sobre O Envelhecimento. 2021;**26**(1)

[71] Tribess S. Prescrição de exercícios físicos para idosos. Saúde.com. 2019;**1**(2):163-172